INTERMITTENT FASTING FOR WOMEN OVER 50

The Complete And Simplified Guide To The Intermittent Fasting Diet For Seniors, To Promote Weight Loss, Health And Longevity

Rosanne Miller

By reading this document, the reader agrees that under no circumstances is the author responsible for any losses, direct or indirect, that are incurred as a result of the use of the information contained within this document, including, but not limited to, errors, omissions, or inaccuracies.

Table of Contents

Introduction

How many diets have you tried in order to lose weight? Let's face it, if you're reading a book like this one, odds are that you feel you need to lose a few pounds to get healthy and feel better. The problem is that losing weight is one of those things that everyone else seems to get right but for some reason, it just doesn't work for you.

I'm here to tell you that losing weight is nowhere near as tough or as difficult as it seems. The reason you've had issues with this is due to poor instruction. That's it! It isn't so much a question of what you've been doing wrong as much as what you haven't been doing right. What I mean is that fancy diets tend to set you up for failure by giving you far too many things to do.

As a result, most people who follow these diets end up spending their time tracking all kinds of things except the ones that really matter. I'm not saying those diets don't work. The ketogenic diet, for example, is a fantastic way to lose fat and get healthier. However, it isn't something you should adopt right off the bat since it can get complicated.

Diets such as keto require you to track calories and calculate your macros. If you have no idea what either of those things are then you're in the right place! The fact is that all of us intuitively know how to eat healthy. You might scoff at this but consider the issue from an evolutionary standpoint. Every species on the planet has a set of built-in mechanisms that allow it to survive and thrive.

Without these mechanisms, human beings would have gone extinct a long time back. The very fact that you've in this world is proof that you have innate skills that will help you live a healthy life. It's just that you've been covering it up with all sorts of bad habits. Our habits are formed thanks to childhood experiences and the sort of environment we grew up in.

In fact, almost every psychological problem we have traces its roots back to issues we encountered in childhood (Morin, 2019). The good news is that these behaviors were learned. What I mean is that if you learned something, you can unlearn it as well. Furthermore, you can install new behaviors within yourself to take the place of those old beliefs and habits.

Doing so requires you to think in new ways and unfortunately, this is where people stumble.

Losing Weight Over 50. Impossible?

When was the last time you tried to make a positive change in your life? It could have been something as simple as waking up earlier or trying to be more productive at work or trying to eat healthier food. Recall how you approached this and whether you were successful or not.

I'm willing to bet any amount of money that in the instances where you made positive changes in your life, you approached your new behaviors in manageable chunks. You didn't try to do too much and simply fell into new behavior. Can you see why your previous diets have been going wrong for you?

When we try to make too many changes all at once, our brains don't react well to this. In fact, they'll do almost anything to reject those changes as quickly as possible. Old habits do indeed die hard. The way to enforce change is to break everything you need to do down into bite-sized pieces and take them on one by one.

Common dieting methods have you implement far too many changes and while you can resort to using your will power to push you through those initial weeks, your brain becomes fatigued and eventually, you're going to give up and go back to what feels comfortable. That is to say, you go back to your old habit patterns.

There's something else your brain does to keep you rooted in your old patterns. It makes up all kinds of beliefs that ensure you don't do anything that might threaten the status quo. Are you someone who believes 50 is too late to be making changes in your life? Do you think that you've lived beyond at least the halfway mark of your life and as such, there's not much more you can do at this point?

This is an example of a limiting belief. The fact is that it is entirely possible to make healthy changes (and unhealthy ones) in your life. You will learn how science proves that age has nothing to do with making changes. The only thing stopping you is your own negative beliefs. Once you understand how they work and where they emerge from, you're going to be in a much better position to make changes.

There's still the issue of trying to figure out what to do in order to enforce positive changes. Is there a method you can adopt that will make it super easy for you to lose weight in a healthy manner and improve your overall health?

Enter Intermittent Fasting

Intermittent fasting, or IF as it's commonly called, is easily the best regime for you to adopt. This is because of how simple it is. In a nutshell, IF dictates that you should fast every day for a certain number of hours and eat solely outside of these fasting hours. That's pretty much it. Sounds simple, doesn't it?

The reason IF works is due to the fact that it is perfectly in line with our natural eating patterns. When left to our own devices, we tend to eat in a pattern that is reminiscent of what IF prescribes. What I mean is that most of us these days tend to eat by the clock or when social settings demand that meals be ingested.

If you were to simply listen to your body and eat only when you feel hungry, you'll find that the number of meals you eat will be low, even if the individual meal size increases slightly. Most of us have divorced ourselves from the signs our bodies give us with regards to hunger and eating and this is why we've come to rely on the clock to tell us when to eat.

IF simplifies all of this and you won't need to worry about following any fancy rules or regulations. Eating itself becomes an easier task because IF removes the need to track and calculate each and every single thing you eat. Of course, if you wish to do this, you're free to do so.

My aim with this book is to not just present this wonderful solution to you, it is also to tell you that your age is just a number. Stop listening to all those voices, including your own, that tell you that it's far too late and that you should simply accept what you've got. You're not a sheep that needs to follow the herd in order to survive.

I'm here to tell you that your goals are not unrealistic at all. If anything, odds are high that you're aiming too low. You'll find that as you make progress, you'll begin to shoot for higher goals. Your goals are entirely up to you. If a certain weight level is your target, then so be it.

If your goal is to make the twenty-somethings at the beach jealous of you, then that's perfectly fine as well. As you read this book, you'll learn how to set goals along with learning the best way of implementing change in your life. Some of the key things that will help you do this are the recipes and the meal plan that I've designed for you.

IF isn't a diet as much as it is a lifestyle. It might sound like hyperbole but IF is the solution you've been looking for all this while for your weight loss issues.

So get ready to embrace change in your life as you head towards your goals! Are you excited yet? Let's get right into it!

Chapter 1:
What is Intermittent Fasting?

Fasting has been practiced by people since ancient times. The reasons for fasting might have varied but almost every ancient culture around the world implemented fasting as a way to improve health and treat disease (Hicks, 2016). A big reason for this is the fact that fasting simplifies a lot of things in our lives when it comes to food and calorie intake.

In this chapter, you're going to learn all about the science behind intermittent fasting and how it works to improve your health. Weight loss is the most visible effect of this lifestyle but its effects go far deeper than that.

The Basics of IF

Intermittent fasting has become increasingly popular in recent times as a lifestyle tool to simplify eating and nutrition. It has been scientifically proven to improve overall health and as a result, people who practice IF tend to live longer (Hicks, 2018). As I mentioned earlier, IF is essentially a cycle that alternates between a fasted state and a feeding state.

In other words, you'll be eating during a certain window while awake and will spend the rest of your time in a fasted state. IF isn't really concerned with what you eat as much as when you eat. This means you're free to eat junk food during your feeding hours but for obvious reasons, you don't want to be doing this.

Eating junk food all the time might not result in weight gain under IF but weight is hardly the sole indicator of overall health. One of the things you must understand is that it is perfectly possible to look thin or lean and be unhealthy on the inside. The flip side is true as well. You need not look super muscular or lean to be healthy.

This doesn't mean an obese person can't be healthy. My point is that health is a holistic thing that goes well beyond how someone looks. It is important for you to understand this fact as it will help you keep your expectations realistic.

As far as the feeding and fasted windows are concerned, their times vary according to the IF method you choose to implement. For example, some methods have you fasting for an entire day while others break the day down into manageable chunks. The next chapter deals with the different types of IF methods so don't worry about this as yet.

In order to understand the benefits of IF, it is important for us to look at how nutrition works at a basic level. Most people do not understand the true function of calories and of hormones such as insulin which play an important role in determining our weight levels.

Furthermore, a lot of people think that exercise is what determines weight levels. While it does have some effect, the fact is that nutrition influences your weight to a far greater degree than exercise does. Let's look at how all of this works.

Nutrients

You are the food you eat. I'm not trying to sound like your mom here but she was right in more ways than one. The food we eat gets turned into all kinds of things once we ingest it and it plays an important role in maintaining the balance of chemicals within our bodies. Broadly speaking, all food is broken down into macronutrients and micronutrients.

Macronutrients are further divided into three types: Fat, carbohydrates, and protein. Fat is often viewed as the enemy when it comes to weight loss. This is an unfortunate result of the language we use. The macronutrient fat is not equivalent to someone being or thinking of themselves as being 'fat.' As such, it has been long misunderstood even in scientific circles.

In fact, for the longest period even the United States Department of Agriculture (USDA) recommended that people minimize the amount of fat they eat in their diets (A Brief History of USDA Food Guides, 2020). Despite this recommendation, obesity rates in America actually soared. It was only in the 90's that the USDA revised its guidelines and admitted that their recommendation had been driven by imperfect research.

It turns out that fat isn't what makes you fat. It is sugar that does so. We'll take a look at sugar in more detail shortly. The primary function of fat is to act as an emergency fuel for your body. Let's say you were dropped in the desert without any food and had to survive. Once your body burned any energy you have stored within you, it will begin to burn fat in order to fuel itself.

An excess of fat is produced in people when their exertion levels are low and their sugar intake is high (How Sugar Converts to Fat, 2020). In fact, when exercise levels are low enough, the body converts almost every single thing ingested into fat because it feels that it needs more in the tank in case an emergency occurs.

Thus, fat levels are not directly influenced by the amount of fat you eat. It's far more complex than that. As such, healthy fats such as the ones found in butter, milk, and cold-pressed oil are essential for our survival. Fats exist in two forms: Saturated and unsaturated.

 Unsaturated fats are necessary for proper bodily functions. As such, they play an important role in heart and brain health (How Sugar Converts to Fat, 2020). Saturated fats are a bit trickier. The fact is that researchers and nutritionists don't fully understand the role they play in our diets. The consensus is that they're needed to a certain degree but an excess of saturated fat is harmful and can lead to terminal diseases like cancer.

This is why the excessive intake of red meat is bad for our health. Red meat contains some of the highest levels of saturated fat which gets converted to cholesterol (the bad type of cholesterol) and ends up clogging our arteries. Excessive levels of saturated fat have been linked to other diseases such as heart disease and stroke (How Sugar Converts to Fat, 2020).

So all in all, fat is good, especially unsaturated fat. As for saturated fat, it is best to minimize it but you shouldn't seek to eliminate it.

The next macronutrient is carbohydrates or carbs. Our old friend sugar is a carb. I'm not trying to say carbs are bad. Much like fat, there isn't a blanket conclusion here. Instead, the levels of carbs are what matter. The USDA recommendation to minimize fat led to an increase in the consumption of carbs in the average American diet.

Coupled with advances in food production technology, this resulted in not just natural carbs but processed carbs being added to our diet as well. Processed foods include chemicals and preservatives that help them last longer. Sugar is a commonly used preservative in such foods and processed sugar is a very different beast from natural sugar that is present in foods such as honey and maple syrup.

Carbs happen to be our bodies' primary fuel source. Going back to the example of being dropped in a desert, your body will first burn all of the carbs that are stored within it. Carbs provide an instant dose of energy and this is why our bodies prefer it. Have you ever eaten a banana prior to working out or exercising and felt a surge of energy?

Bananas are a major source of carbs and when burned by the body, those carbs are converted to glucose which is burned by the body to produce energy. Glucose by itself doesn't produce energy. Instead, it is converted to energy by insulin, which is a hormone that is secreted by an organ called the Pancreas (Cotton, 2019).

People who suffer from diabetes have low levels of insulin in their bloodstream. As a result, glucose remains in the bloodstream and isn't burned. Similarly, if you were to consume excessive levels of carbs, the body leaves the excess glucose as it is since it simply doesn't need it.

This excess has to be stored somewhere and the body decides to convert it to fat. Thus, excessive consumption of carbs leads to additional fat being stored in your body. A malfunctioning pancreas in people who suffer from diabetes makes them extremely sensitive to carb intake. This is why the ketogenic diet, which is a diet that advocates eating high levels of fat and low carbs, helps curb the adverse effects of diabetes.

I'm not advocating eating low levels of carbs (unless you're diabetic.) It's just that you need to eat the right amount and make sure there aren't too many excess carbs floating around in your system. Carbs are a great source of energy and are in fact essential to getting stronger. They help fuel your workouts and as a result, people who are looking to build muscle are advised to eat more carbs.

The muscle mass of your body is a measure of how strong you are. Simply put, the more muscle you have, the greater your ability to withstand adverse conditions. If two people, one with low muscle mass and another with high levels of it, were dropped in a desert, the person with high muscle mass would be able to sustain themselves for longer. Their body will delay the burning of emergency fat since they have enough strength to get by. This doesn't mean they're superhuman. It's just that they're more likely to fare better than the other person.

Your muscles are made of protein which happens to be the third macronutrient. While the body has two sources of energy in carbs and fat, the fact is that it has just one source of muscle. This means you need to eat protein with every meal to feed your muscles. This doesn't mean you should eat just protein. Remember, protein is not an energy source.

If you were to eat high levels of protein and low levels of fat and carbs, you'll feed your muscles but they won't have any fuel to power them. Think of the situation as being akin to building a huge spaceship but not having any fuel to power the thing. It isn't of much use is it?

Common advice is to eat between 0.7-1g of protein per pound of bodyweight. IF doesn't require you to count calories but protein intake is essential and as such, you should track this at a bare minimum. This isn't very hard to do and you'll learn how to incorporate this into your life easily in later chapters.

For now, keep this in mind: You need to eat protein in adequate amounts. You're free to eat more but remember that you'll end up reducing your fat and carb intake by doing so and this is unhealthy. As for fat and carbs, choose to maximize one and minimize the other. Since both are sources of fuel for your body, you can theoretically eliminate one of them completely.

For the reasons for eating a balanced diet, this is not recommended. However, you can minimize one macronutrient. The ketogenic diet is an example of minimizing carbs while maximizing fat. If the idea of that appeals to you, go for it. However, if you've never implemented a diet successfully enough to see results, I recommend minimizing fat and maximizing carbs.

By maximizing, I don't mean load up on carbs. Eat as you normally would and become more aware of what you're eating. For example, if you're eating a plate of pasta with creamy alfredo sauce and bacon, you're not getting enough protein (just bacon) and are in fact eating high levels of carbs (pasta) and fat (sauce and bacon.)

So what does all of this have to do with weight loss?

How Weight Loss Works

All macronutrients contribute calories to your body. Everyone needs a base amount of calories to function. You can think of calories as fuel. Just as every vehicle needs some level of fuel to work, so do you need calories to function to a certain degree.

If you eat an amount of calories that is greater than what you need, your body is going to convert those calories to muscle or fat and store it as such. If you were to eat less, your body is going to burn muscle or fat to make up for the deficit (Scott, 2019). Hence, if you were to eat less, you will lose weight. Notice that your body can burn either fat or muscle.

This is why there's an unhealthy and healthy way to lose weight. If you were to lose muscle, you're actually losing strength and your body is going to compensate by increasing the level of fat in your body. Thus, you'll lose weight to a certain point and then simply put on more fat. You'll be at a lower body weight but will look fatter than you were. Obviously, this is not what we're after.

There is another problem with restricting calories. The fact is that our bodies are extremely intelligent and can adapt to pretty much any circumstance, within reason. If you restrict calories for too long, your body's metabolism decreases. In other words, it will shut down certain non-essential faculties and will seek to get by on less energy.

It will also get you to expend less energy and as a result, your weight loss will plateau. All of this places a strain on you, both physically and mentally, and you'll never achieve your goals. This is how most diets play out. They work for a while but the minute the body's metabolism drops, they stop working because the body has adjusted and the deficit has no effect anymore.

This is where IF differs from the rest. For one thing, you can eat whatever you want. Obviously, it is best to eat a balanced diet that is rich in protein (as per the recommended amount) and high in either fat or carbs. Second, your feeding window is curtailed. In other words, you'll be eating in a smaller time window than usual and as a result, you'll be eating when hungry.

This means your body is in a prime position to convert the calories you eat into muscle and your fat gains will be minimal. Another effect of restricting meal times is that you'll automatically eat the right portion sizes for you. After all, there's only so much a person can eat in a single sitting.

During the fasted state, your body will have to figure out how to get its nutrition and as a result, it will burn the excess carbs and fat in your body. It might burn muscle as well but you'll learn how to prevent this later in this book. The bottom line is that IF will help you lose weight in a healthy manner without needing you to make massive changes.

All you have to do is eat within specified intervals as you normally would and track your protein intake. That's it! If you follow healthy eating guidelines, you'll manage to ensure you achieve your goals and improve your health overall.

Micronutrients

While macronutrients have three types within them, there are a large number of micronutrients. These can be broadly classified as being vitamins and minerals. All of them are needed in some quantity to ensure your body works optimally.

You might be wondering how on earth can you ensure you're eating the right quantity of micronutrients? This is where a balanced diet comes into play. A balanced diet is one that contains a good degree of diversity within it. Diversity refers to both macronutrient profile as well as things such as texture and color.

Creating a balanced diet is not as hard as you think. What does the color of the food on your plate look like? Balanced diets have variety in them in more ways than one! Meat and fat heavy plates tend to acquire a brown or white tinge. Adding some green and red on there makes sure you'll consume your ideal share of vegetables.

Leafy green vegetables happen to be some of the best sources of micronutrients. In addition to this, you can also supplement them. I'll address supplements in a separate chapter. For now, just keep in mind that as long as your diet is balanced, you'll receive your share of micronutrients.

Sources of Macronutrients

You might be wondering which foods are the best sources of carbs, protein, and fat? This section is going to give you a good idea of what sort of nutrient profile most foods have. Let's begin by looking at sources of carbs.

Carbs

Generally speaking all kinds of grains, foods derived from grains such as pasta (flour) and vegetables are great sources of carbs. Fruits are also high in carbs, with the exception of avocado which is high in fat and protein and is low in carbs. The primary source of carbs in fruits is sugar.

Keep in mind that the sugar found in fruits is not the sort of harmful processed sugar you find in junk food. Having said that, it's not a good idea to load up on fruits all the time if you're looking to lose weight since you can easily consume excess carbs ("Is The Sugar in Fruit Wrecking Your Diet?", 2020). The rate of your fat gain won't be large but those excess carbs will need to be stored somewhere.

Here is a handy and healthy list of carb-heavy foods:

- Whole grains
    - Brown/Red/Black/Wild rice
    - Wheat/Bulgur/Cracked wheat
    - Quinoa
    - Couscous
- Vegetables
    - Potatoes
    - Sweet potatoes
    - Beans
        - Kidney
        - Black
        - Brown
        - White
    - Chickpeas/Garbanzo beans
    - Carrots
    - Peas
    - Leafy green vegetables
        - Spinach
        - Kale
        - Lettuce
        - Cabbage (red cabbage as well)
    - Beets/Beetroot
    - Turnips
    - Eggplants
    - Onions

- Fruits
  - Bananas
  - Apples
  - Pears
  - Pineapples
  - Mangoes
  - Oranges
- Lentils

When it comes to carbs, you'll read a lot about something called fiber. In short, fiber is what ensures your colon remains clean and that all the waste within it gets flushed. Vegetables and fruits (especially leafy greens and fibrous fruits like oranges) are high in fiber and you should eat a healthy serving of these.

The best way to tell if you're eating enough fiber is to look at the quality of your stools. As long as you can comfortably pass them, you're eating a decent quantity of fiber.

Fat

Even if you're looking to minimize fat in your diet you're going to end up consuming some form of it. Don't worry too much about reducing your fat intake and maximizing carbs on IF. Once you've gained some experience with the diet, you'll be able to figure out roughly how much fat and carbs you're consuming comparatively speaking.

Generally speaking, dairy and oils happen to be high in fat. In addition to this, there are certain foods that are known to be high in other macronutrients but contain high levels of fat as well. Here is a brief list of healthy fat sources.

- Cold-pressed oils
    - Extra virgin olive oil
    - Coconut oil
    - Rice bran oil
- Butter
- Whole milk (especially cow's milk)
- Nuts
    - Almonds
    - Sunflower seeds
    - Walnut
- Cream
    - Cooking cream
    - Whipped cream
- Ghee/clarified butter

Nuts make for a healthy snack but it is possible to eat too much fat when consuming them since they're extremely calorie-dense. In other words, they pack a huge number of calories in a small package.

Protein

Given its importance, you should familiarize yourself with the list of protein sources. Broadly speaking, all forms of meat are extremely dense in protein. This makes sense because meat is essentially animal muscle. White meat such as chicken breast and turkey happen to be high in protein and low in fat and carbs.

Red meat such as beef and pork is high in protein and high in saturated fat as well. When consuming red meat, you should choose leaner cuts to minimize your fat intake. Given that this is saturated fat, you should be conscious of how much red meat you consume.

Fish and seafood happen to be great sources of protein. Oily fish such as sardines and mackerel are excellent sources of both protein and fat. In fact, canned sardines are some of the best sources of protein you can find off the shelf in your supermarket. The issue with fish is that as you move up the food chain, you're more likely to find greater concentrations of what is referred to as mercury.

This is a blanket term for the amount of pollution the fish ingests. Bigger fish such as marlin, tuna, and salmon not only consume the pollution inherent in the water they swim in but also through the smaller fish they eat. Thus, you should minimize the consumption of these kinds of fish, no matter how delicious they might be.

Here is a brief list of great protein sources, including vegetarian ones.

- Meat
    - Chicken breast
    - Chicken thighs/dark meat (these contain more fat)
    - Beef (high in saturated fat)
    - Pork (high in saturated fat)
    - Turkey
    - Any other wild/game meat (usually high in fat with exceptions)
- Fish and seafood
    - Sardines
    - Tuna
    - Salmon
    - Mackerel
    - Shrimp
    - Lobster
    - Crab
    - Trout/Bass etc
- Tofu
- Tempeh
- Chickpeas
- Beans
- Lentils

When it comes to vegetarian protein sources, you must keep in mind that these are carb-heavy. You will often see food like chickpeas being touted as being protein-heavy but the fact is that they have higher levels of carbs. This doesn't make them bad. It's just that you need to be aware of this fact.

Animal-based sources tend to have high levels of protein and are low in everything else. Red meat, which is considered high in saturated fat, actually has more protein than fat in terms of grams. Thus, the term 'protein-heavy' is relative and you should pay attention to the other nutrients present.

Generally speaking, chicken breast, turkey and fish are the only foods that have protein almost exclusively.

The Benefits of IF

There are a number of benefits to IF and in this section, you're going to learn about some of them. One of the biggest benefits that occur is that in the fasted state, your body adjusts its hormone levels in order to make stored fat more accessible (Coyle, 2018). This is because the body initiates repair and recovery processes while fasted and this affects hormone levels in the body.

Hormonal Levels

The first hormone that increases in level is HGH or human growth hormone. Some studies have measured the increase to be as much as fivefold (Coyle, 2018). Increased levels of HGH have been linked to fat loss and muscle gain.

Insulin levels also dramatically drop when fasted. Remember that the presence of insulin in the bloodstream is a signal for the body to burn glucose. As long as insulin is present, your body fat will not be accessible since it will not be prioritized as a fuel source. Your body becomes more sensitive to insulin levels when fasted and as a result, the levels of it in your bloodstream drops faster.

In addition to these two, other effects have been observed which affect gene expression. This in turn affects longevity and the immune system (Coyle, 2018).

Autophagy

Autophagy refers to a cellular process where repair processes are initiated. During this time, harmful proteins that build up within them are ejected and your cells essentially rejuvenate themselves (Coyle, 2018).

This process always takes place in a fasted state and thanks to the regime imposed by IF, autophagy takes place for longer and occurs more efficiently. In essence, your cells clean themselves more efficiently and for longer.

Inflammation

Inflammation is your body's response to any adverse physical circumstances. For example, if you are physically injured, the injured area is inflamed to enable a faster healing response.

The problem with inflammation is that when it becomes chronic, your body is placed under a lot of stress that affects its functions adversely (Coyle, 2018).

Studies have shown that intermittent fasting reduces the occurrence of inflammation and this, in turn, reduces the occurrence of chronic diseases.

Heart Health

Thanks to the body's increased insulin sensitivity, IF when combined with a healthy and balanced diet can reduce the risk of suffering heart disease. This is the result of bad cholesterol being reduced significantly. Bad cholesterol, or LDL as it's called (as opposed to HDL which is good cholesterol,) is what clogs your arteries and increases the risk of a heart attack.

When your body becomes more insulin sensitive, greater amounts of fat are burned and as a result, the levels of saturated fat decrease. Mind you, this doesn't mean you can eat any amount of saturated fat and expect IF to burn it automatically. A balanced diet is what ensures this happens during the fasted state.

Extended Lifespan

While this hasn't been proved in human beings as yet, studies conducted on lab rats show an increase in lifespan of up to 80%. The point here is that if a rat can benefit from IF, chances are it will have some effect on you as well. Given the numerous health benefits, this isn't such a stretch to believe.

Brain Health

In addition to improving heart health, IF also increases the brain hormone BDNF which aids the growth of new cells. This, in turn, helps reduce the risk of dementia and Alzheimer's disease (Coyle, 2018).

Risks For Women

Despite the huge health benefits that IF brings to those who practice it, there are indications that it might not be as beneficial for women as it is for men. A study that measured blood sugar levels amongst both men and women showed that insulin sensitivity amongst women actually got worse while it got better for men (Coyle, 2018).

There is speculation that these kinds of results have nothing to do with IF by itself but are instead a reflection of the fact that women are more sensitive to dietary changes and fasting than men are as a group. This view is backed up by anecdotal evidence of women experiencing changes in their menstrual cycles upon changing their diet.

The key to understand is that everything circles around calorie intake. Research shows that women are far more sensitive to reduced calorie intakes than men are. Long fasting periods place a lot of pressure in this regard and this is why certain forms of IF might not be suited for women.

The best approach for women appears to be to utilize smaller fasting windows than men and to ensure that their calorie intake remains high. This doesn't mean you need to track your calories minutely. It's just that you need to listen to your body and what it tells you.

Contrary to popular perception, you should not feel high levels of hunger when fasting. Most people think that this is some sort of indication that IF is working when really, it's your body telling you that you're not eating enough calories. If this happens to you, feel free to break your fast and have a small meal.

In addition to this, you should not practice IF if you have had any of the following occur to you:

- Eating disorders
- Diabetes
- If you are underweight currently
- Are pregnant or trying to conceive
- Have fertility problems
- Have experienced amenorrhea (missed periods)

After beginning IF, monitor yourself for any adverse symptoms and watch out for any missed menstrual cycles or changes to it. If this happens, contact your doctor and check with them to see if continuing IF is advisable for you.

Despite all of this don't mistake IF as being something extremely risky for women or for someone of your age. As I mentioned earlier, the changes you need to make aren't huge and generally speaking very few people have issues with this lifestyle.

Chapter 2:
The Types of Intermittent Fasting

While the basic premise of IF is simple, there are many different ways of putting it into action. The method you choose depends on your lifestyle and other factors that influence your eating habits. What some people might find easy to follow might not be practical for others.

This chapter is going to help you choose the best method for you to follow along with helping you learn all the different ways in which IF can be implemented.

Daily, Time Based Approaches

There are a number of methods that differentiate themselves on the basis of the size of their fasting and feeding windows. Technically this is true for every method in this chapter but these particular methods follow a daily fasting and feeding schedule.

The most common approach is the so called 16:8 where people fast for 16 hours a day and eat within an eight-hour window. This might seem like a long fasting window but consider that your time spent sleeping is a part of the fasting window. Assuming you sleep for eight hours, this means you'll be eating over an eight hour period and fasting while awake for another eight. That doesn't seem so bad, does it?

There are other ratios you could follow such as 14:10, 20:4, 12:12 and Leangains. I'll dive into Leangains shortly but with the other approaches, your sleeping time is incorporated into the fasting period. Some are more extreme than others. For example, a split of 20:4 is not advisable for women due to the issues presented in the previous chapter.

A split of 14:10 might be the most convenient when starting out. The key thing to keep in mind is that all of these methods require you to eat as you normally would during your feeding window. Don't think of this time as you being given a free license to binge or eat any amounts of junk food.

If your diet needs fixing, follow this simple method. Make the base of all of your meals whole grains as listed in the previous chapter. Incorporate some form of protein in appropriate quantities and add leafy greens and some vegetables and fruits. What is an 'appropriate' amount of protein? As mentioned earlier, your daily intake should be around 0.7-1 gram of protein per pound of bodyweight. For example, if you weigh 150 lbs, you should be eating between 105-150 grams of protein every day. Divide this number by the number of meals you have and you'll figure out how much protein you need to eat.

Do not use any cooking oils other than the ones mentioned in the list of healthy fats. Once you clean your diet in this manner, you will become healthier automatically. From that point onwards, it's just a question of maintaining your diet regime.

None of these time-based approaches need you to do anything special other than following the fasting and feeding windows. The only exception to this is Leangains

Leangains

Leangains is a program developed by the Swedish nutritionist and powerlifter Martin Berkhan (Leangains.com, 2020). As such Berkhan was one of the first people to tout the benefits of intermittent fasting and Leangains remains one of the most popular forms of implementing IF to this day.

As such, the program doesn't have any specific stipulations. This is due to the fact that Berkhan designs programs for his clients as their needs might be. Obviously, you will need to become his client and pay his fees to have him design a diet and protocols for you. The effectiveness of Leangains is borne out by the fact that there is a substantial waiting list for Berkhan's services.

Despite all of this, there are quite a few clues Berkhan has mentioned over the years on the Leangains website. For starters, it appears that he advocates easing into the program by selecting longer feeding windows. This means a feeding window of 10 or eight hours is appropriate for most beginners.

A 10-hour feeding window implies six hours of fasting (assuming you'll sleep for eight hours) while awake.

This is a normal day for most people and will not impact your schedule too much. The ideal fasting and feeding split would be 16:8 since the eight hours you will spend fasted awake will force your body to change and burn additional fat.

Leangains is a fat loss program at heart and given Berkhan's background, it is designed for bodybuilders. As a result, there is a huge emphasis placed on working out with heavy, compound lifts. Over the years, anecdotal evidence suggests that it isn't the lifts themselves that are important in this method but rather the intensity of exercise.

Berkhan divides Leangains' goals into three categories:

1. Losing fat
2. Body recomposition
3. Gaining muscles

The first objective is realized by maintaining a caloric deficit. As I mentioned in the previous chapter, you need not follow this since women are far more sensitive to reduced caloric intake than men are.

The second objective is what you'll shoot for. In this regime, you'll eat as much as you need to in order to maintain your current weight. The combination of fasting plus high-intensity workouts will mean that you will replace fat with muscle.

However, there is a catch with this, and indeed all of Leangains.

You will need to calculate your macros and track them accurately. Furthermore, since macro calculation is a trial and error process, you will need to make frequent changes to the food you eat in terms of quantity. As such, since this approach involves making a lot of changes at once, it is appropriate to follow if you have someone like Berkhan or a trainer who can advise you and hold you accountable.

If not, a good alternative is to adopt the Leangains approach to a traditional 16:8 diet (or any other time partition that makes sense to you). The primary rule of Leangains that you will borrow has to do with workout intensity. I'll go into workouts in more detail in a later chapter. For now, understand that you will need to hit the gym for the best results.

"What if I don't want to hit the gym and still want all the great results?" you might be thinking. This is a bit like wanting someone to write you a check for any amount of money you want but not wanting to do the work to earn that paycheck. It's a bit unrealistic. You need to be physically active and push yourself in order to ensure that you don't put on more fat and instead replace your existing fat with muscle.

A wrinkle that Berkhan adds in this regime is that during non-workout days, you should eat higher levels of fat and on workout days, you should minimize fat and maximize carbs. In essence, on non-workout days you should follow the keto diet for all intents and purposes while you follow a high carb diet on workout days.

Following this will require you to count calories and macros and if this doesn't appeal to you, there's no need for you to do so. As I mentioned, it's best to apply the Leangains workout principle to a common 16:8 partition and work from there.

There are a few other nuances regarding workouts that I will cover in the chapter dealing with them. Since these tips apply to every IF method, it makes sense to split it out into a full chapter. If you do wish to follow Leangains to the T, my recommendation would be to gather some experience with IF prior to trying to do it all by yourself.

This is because counting calories and macros is not a straightforward task. However, in the interest of presenting all the information with regards to Leangains, I will address this. Those of you who do not wish to count calories can safely skip ahead to the section after the following one.

Counting Calories

As I mentioned earlier, weight loss or gain is a function of calories eaten versus calories expended. If the former is greater than the latter, you will put on weight. Since your objective here is to recompose your body, you will eat at what is called the maintenance level. In other words, you'll eat as much as you need or even eat at a slight excess.

Counting calories is of no use unless you back it up with a heavy workout, so make sure you review the information in that chapter once you're done with this. To count calories, we begin first by figuring out our necessary caloric intake.

This number is referred to as the Basal Metabolic Rate or BMR. The most common method of calculating the BMR is to use either the Mifflin-St Jeor equation or the Harris-Benedict formula. There are subtle differences between both but overall for our purposes, they spit out pretty much the same number.

The best way of calculating this number is to use the calculator at https://www.calculator.net/bmr-calculator.html or you can search online for one yourself. The following factors influence your BMR:

4. Age
5. Height
6. Sex
7. Weight
8. Activity level

Plug your information into the calculator and adjust it for your activity level. The activity level refers to how physically active you are and this is usually a place where most people go wrong. They tend to overestimate their activity levels grossly.

A good rule of thumb when first counting calories is to assume a sedentary activity level and then readjust your numbers as time goes on.

Once you receive your BMR number, this is your caloric target. Now, you need to figure out your macro partitions. We first begin by calculating the amount of protein we need to eat.

As I mentioned earlier, this is pretty simple. You multiply your body weight in pounds by any number from 0.7 to one and this gives you the number of grams of protein you need to eat. Next, multiply that number by four. The result is the number of calories released by eating protein.

For example, let's say your BMR is 2000 calories and your body weight is 150lbs.

Protein intake = 150*1gram/lb = 150 g
Calories from protein = 150*4 cal/gram = 600

This means we need to divide the remaining (2000-600 = 1400) 1,400 calories between carbs and fat. We're looking at minimizing fat and maximizing carbs. Thus, let's assume that 80% of these remaining calories come from carbs.

In other words, calories from carbs = 1,120 calories

Carbs release four calories per gram. Dividing 1,120 by four gives us 280 grams of carbs.

Amount of carbs to eat = Total calories from carbs/calories per gram from carbs = 1120/4 = 280g

We do the same thing to figure out calories from fat. We know that 20% of 1,400 calories come from fat. Hence,

Calories from fat = 1400*.2 = 280

Amount of fat to eat = Total calories from fat/calories per gram from fat = 280/8 = 35g

Hence, our final macro breakdown is:

Protein = 150g
Carbs = 280g
Fat = 35g

If you wish, you could increase carb intake even further and reduce fat intake. If you want to follow the keto diet, once you've figured out calories from protein, you will need to minimize carbs instead of minimizing fat as we did here. In other words, set 80-90% of your remaining calories as coming from fat (instead of carbs as we did here.)

Once this is done, all you'll need to do is plug your food into a calculator and figure out how much of something you need to eat. It's best to use online software such as the ones at Fitday or Cronometer that will automatically give you the calorie and macro numbers for foods.

This will be your food list and you can create meals from this list as you wish. An important thing for you to do is to adjust your caloric intake as you go along. You will need to track your body weight and if you find that you're gaining weight or are losing weight on a week by week basis, you will need to decrease or increase your caloric intake by around 250 calories.

Once you land on the right number, keep eating the same amounts of food and keep working out hard in the gym and you'll begin to see changes over time. Typically, it will take three months for you to see any changes in the mirror.

If you want to follow the full Leangains protocol, you will need to cycle carbs. In other words, during your workout days you'll maximize carbs and on non-workout days, you'll maximize fat. As such, you'll have two macro partitions to keep track of and different diets on both days.

This is a bit more complicated as you can imagine but Berkhan's success proves that it is the most effective method of fat loss. It takes work of course but the results are well worth it. Make sure you read the chapter on exercise to make sure you understand how the method works fully.

The Warrior Diet

As the name suggests, the Warrior diet doesn't do things half baked. It's origin story lives up to its name as well. Developed by an Israeli special forces soldier turned nutritionist, Ori Hofmekler, this diet is perhaps the most extreme form of IF you can follow.

The premise of the diet has nothing to do with IF, in reality. Hofmekler openly admits that his diet is not grounded in or based on any scientific research. Instead, his aim was to bring the diet of an ancient warrior to the mainstream. As such, the plans in the diet are based on Hofmekler's own beliefs. It is a coincidence that his prescriptions happen to fit into an IF framework and this is why the Warrior diet is considered a part of IF.

The idea, according to Hofmekeler, is to trigger the body's survival instincts and thus help it perform a lot better. The diet itself places a lot of stress on the body by requiring several hours of undereating and four concentrated hours of binge eating. In other words, the fasting window is 20 hours long and the feeding window lasts for four hours (Kubala, 2018).

Technically, the 20-hour window isn't a fasting window since dieters are encouraged to eat small amounts of food during this time. Typical recommendations include a small amount of fruit or dairy along with lots of water and coffee to keep energy levels up. Given how extreme this diet is, there is an initiation plan which dieters are recommended to put themselves through in order to be able to successfully transition into it.

Week One

The first week is labeled the detox week. During this time, dieters should consume dairy, hard-boiled eggs, vegetable juices, and clear broth during the 20-hour window. Once the four-hour window starts, dieters should consume a large salad followed by large meals of plant-based proteins, cheese, and whole grains.

In addition to this, drinks such as coffee, tea and water can be consumed throughout the day.

Week Two

The second week is dubbed the high-fat phase and during this time, dieters should aim to consume zero grains or starch. The advice to consume broth, dairy and fruits during the fasting period applies here as well.

During the feeding phase, Hofmekeler mentions that the only source of protein should be lean animal protein along with substantial servings of cooked vegetables and cheese.

Week Three

The third week gets a little more complicated. During this time, you will cycle your carbs and will dedicate two days of the week to consuming high amounts of carbs and three days to high fat. Protein remains high all throughout. The usual rules regarding what to eat when fasting and having high amounts of both plant and animal-based protein apply (Kubala, 2018).

Once the three weeks are done, dieters can either follow the same cycle again or simply follow a plan where they consume high protein meals during the four-hour window with large servings of cooked vegetables.

Guidelines

One of the knocks against the warrior diet is that it lacks any sort of caloric guidelines for dieters. The only rule mentioned is that dieters should avoid processed foods and sugar such as candy. Fried foods and junk food are also not allowed and all meals must be constructed from whole food sources.

In addition to this, fruit juices are also not allowed since these contain high amounts of sugar. You can consume fruits by themselves or have vegetable juices.

Advantages and Disadvantages

Given that the warrior diet isn't something that is based on scientific fact, there isn't a huge body of research that has been carried out on it. Generally speaking, researchers argue that the benefits of the diet mirror that of an IF diet. Given the small feeding window, it is almost impossible to binge eat on this diet and this results in some form of weight control automatically.

When viewed in this frame, it makes sense that there are no caloric guidelines since it would only put further strain on the dieters. Instead, the regime puts a dieter in better touch with her hunger and instincts and this has a number of advantages when it comes to undoing the effects of the clock on hunger and overeating.

Unhealthy habits such as snacking on chips and other fried foods are also eliminated. One of the downsides is that there is no strict definition for what qualifies as undereating during the 20-hour block. While dieters are allowed to have vegetable juices, it is possible to consume a lot of calories from this and dairy products.

It can be difficult for beginner dieters to have the discipline to refrain from eating too much during this period when hunger strikes. As a result, the impact of the four-hour feeding window is dulled and the dieter might end up eating too much. The windows themselves are pretty extreme and not everyone will be able to follow its prescriptions.

After all, undereating for 20 hours is tough, 12 of which will be spent awake. Given that there is just a four-hour feeding window, how a dieter can incorporate this into their social lives is a tough question to answer. I mean, you could order the entire menu when out at a restaurant but that will likely earn you a few stares.

Lastly, given the strain this diet places on the body, very few women will likely find this suited for them. The hormonal swings and potential side effects might be too adverse and you must consult your doctor before adopting this diet.

5:2 Diet

While the warrior diet was developed by a special forces soldier, this diet was developed by a journalist. As of this writing, the 5:2 diet or 5/2 as it's sometimes referred to, is the most popular IF diet out there. Like the warrior diet, it's roots don't necessarily lie in IF but its rules fit very well into the protocol.

In terms of rules, the diet is pretty simple to follow. You eat normally for five days of the week and designate two days to severely restrict calories. The two days should not be consecutive. For men, the number of calories to consume on the two days is 600 and this number is 500 for women.

During the three days, you eat as you normally would and don't restrict what you're eating. The only advice provided here is to consume as many unprocessed whole foods as possible. Other than this, there is no need to cycle your macros or even count them in any shape or form.

Typically people choose to consume three meals with a snack during the five days. During the calorie-restricted days, you can choose to spread the meager calorie count throughout the day or have a single meal account for it all.

Advantages and Disadvantages

Given that the rules are so straightforward, the diet can be adopted by pretty much anyone. There is no requirement to exercise but it is recommended that you pursue some level of activity. As I mentioned earlier, the diet itself doesn't derive from IF principles but ends up mimicking it anyway.

Thus, the benefits that you would realize from following a typical IF diet will be replicated here. There are however some drawbacks. While the lack of rigid guidelines helps people adopt the diet easily, they are also a disadvantage. The very reason people adopt diets is due to the fact that they're not used to eating in a healthy or controlled manner.

Put another way, most would-be dieters have a poor idea of how much food is enough and aren't fully in touch with their sense of hunger. To advise these people to eat as they normally would for five days of the week might not be the best advice out there (Kubala, 2018). It is true that calories are severely restricted for two days of the week but on the day after the restriction ends, people are more likely to binge eat.

The lack of guidelines as to what to eat on non-restricted days will make the binge eating potentially worse. Also, people might feel the need to overeat prior to a restricted day in an effort to somehow 'store' calories. These issues aren't really addressed by the diet.

The other issue is that restricting calories all of a sudden has a bunch of side effects such as weakness, dizziness and so on. The protocol is to consider this normal and to adjust to this within a week. If these symptoms persist, the diet should be dropped. It seems excessive to suffer through dizziness and weak spells as a norm before you can figure out whether it is for you.

All in all, despite the ease of adoption, the 5:2 is a diet that does a few things well but falls short of the benefits of other protocols such as a daily limited diet or even the warrior diet which has a rigid discipline to it. It offers the general illusion of discipline but falls short on many counts.

The biggest shortfall is the fat loss plateau you will encounter once your body adjusts to the new regime. It will simply store more fat prior to a restricted day and your weight will remain at roughly the same level throughout the time you follow the diet.

Eat, Stop, Eat

Eat stop eat was developed by Brad Pilon and is a more disciplined take on the 5/2 diet. Pilon is a bodybuilder himself and the diet he's developed reflects this. While the 5/2 limits calories on certain days, eat stop eat eliminates them entirely. Thus, you will be fasting for a full 24 hour period twice a week.

Like with 5/2, these days will be non-consecutive. While there aren't any restrictions placed on what you should eat during the five feeding days, Pilon does provide plenty of guidance as to what to eat. Besides, the fact that you will be fasting for 48 hours per week will cause a greater caloric deficit and will hence aid weight loss to a greater degree.

Pilon designed this diet to conform to the IF protocol and as a result, this diet is scientifically proven to match the benefits that IF provides. In addition to this, there are many other advantages.

Advantages and Disadvantages

The presence of a strong framework and guidelines with regards to what to eat is perhaps the biggest advantage eat stop eat has over the 5/2 diet. Given Pilon's background, you're also ensured that advice comes from a trusted and authoritative source.

While the fasting periods will be tough to handle initially, Pilon provides helpful guidelines to manage these periods. You will feel the same initial side effects as the 5/2 and there's no way to avoid this, unfortunately. Furthermore, the exact link between this diet and weight loss has not been fully established via research (Kubala, 2018).

Thus, there is the danger that the protocol might work for some but not for others. The presence of the two 24 hour windows might be too extreme for some people and it is likely that this will trigger some hormonal changes in women.

The best way to evaluate it is to check with your doctor to see if this is suitable for you to follow.

Alternate Day Fasts

While eat stop eat has you fasting for 24-hour windows twice a week, ADF or Alternate Day Fasts has you skipping meals for 36 hours. As such, there isn't much of a difference in terms of fasting versus feeding protocol between ADF and the rest of the methods we've looked at thus far.

Generally speaking, you need to eat high levels of protein and avoid junk food. Design your meals from whole food sources and make sure your diet is balanced. As always, hydration is key and you should monitor yourself for dehydration, especially on fasting days.

The advantages of ADF are similar to eat stop eat and it also shares the same disadvantages. It might be too extreme for some people and the abrupt switches between eating fully and not eating at all might cause adverse hormonal changes in some.

All in all, you should consult your doctor prior to committing to any method that has you fasting for an entire day.

Spontaneous Meal Skipping

Historically speaking, human beings never had constant access to food like we do these days. As a result, our ancestors developed a strong connection between their sense of hunger and their brains. The abundance of food in the western world these days has led us to adopt a three meals a day eating pattern.

This has led us to believe that skipping a meal has adverse consequences and that it is something that should be avoided at all costs. As I mentioned earlier, this is the clock effect we follow when it comes to our meal times. We often eat simply because it is time to do so and not because we're hungry.

Spontaneous meal skipping comes from the eating philosophy termed intuitive eating. This isn't really a protocol as much as it is an admonishment to simply listen to your body when the time comes to eat. This might sound as if there are zero rules and technically there are no rules when it comes to this.

However, it is still a great regime to follow since it puts you back in touch with your natural instincts for hunger. There are times when we eat too much in a single sitting and don't really need a full meal when the time for it comes. During such moments, it is best to simply skip the meal or to eat a smaller meal.

This is what spontaneous meal skipping is all about. By simply listening to your body, you will develop healthy eating habits. You might argue that the 5/2 method has a similar lack of rules but I wasn't in favor of that protocol. The reason for this contradiction is that the 5/2 method imposes the illusion of rules by specifying enforced low-calorie periods. You might find that a low-calorie day might not suit what your body is telling you.

Spontaneous meal skipping, on the other hand, doesn't have such issues. The only downside is that it will take time to get used to listening to your body and you might not see huge results for a while. Besides, the ultimate aim of this protocol is to put you in a better state of mind with regard to your body image and how you feel about yourself.

It isn't necessarily geared towards losing weight or fat so if that's what you're looking for, spontaneous meal skipping is not for you. Generally speaking, it is a great protocol to adopt once you've reached your goal and wish to maintain your current levels of health. Your body will get used to being at this healthier state and will know what it needs to nourish itself.

The benefits of skipping meals spontaneously are more mental than physical. There isn't a large body of research that has been conducted on this method and as I mentioned, its aim is to improve your relationship with food and reduce the adversarial nature of mind versus hunger.

Crescendo Fasting

Crescendo fasting combines the benefits of all the methods we've looked at thus far into one easily manageable protocol which is perhaps the best suited for women. It is also the one that can be adopted the most easily by beginners to IF. Briefly, here's how it works.

You implement IF for two days a week on non-consecutive days. This means on two days of the week, you will be fasting for 16 hours a day and will be eating within an eight-hour window. Once your body adjusts to this cycle, you can add a third non-consecutive day to your routine.

As you can see, the Crescendo method is a great way to ease yourself into the world of intermittent fasting. There is no need for you to go hungry for entire days on end and you don't need to worry at first about having to go hungry for extended periods every single day. It is also a great way for you to ease into IF since you won't be fasting every single day and your body will have time to adjust to the new situation.

Given that you will be fasting intermittently on non-consecutive days, you will gain the full benefits of IF as listed previously. While you will not see the same rate of fat loss as you would with a regular 16/8 or Leangains protocol (or a modified 16/8 with Leangains method as detailed earlier in this chapter,) you will notice the benefits over time.

Perhaps the biggest advantage of the Crescendo method is that it will stop you from sabotaging yourself. As I mentioned in the introduction, one of the reasons diets fail is that they seek to implement far too many changes over a short period of time. Our brains simply cannot handle that much change and as a result, we end up breaking our rules and undoing all the progress we made.

This danger is removed with the Crescendo method since you're not rushing into anything. You begin with two IF days, add a third and as you'll see in the next chapter, this puts you in a prime position to make even more progress when it comes to implementing IF fully.

Another reason diets fail is that they tend to make us fall foul of social obligations. Imagine having to attend a dinner with friends and having a bunch of insane dietary requirements or simply not eating anything. Most people prefer to avoid such situations and the Crescendo method preempts all of this in a simple method.

All in all, this method is the best one for you to adopt if you're unsure about your ability to stick to a diet or lifestyle over the long term. If you're a bit more confident, the modified 16/8 method will work well for you.

This brings us nicely to our next point, which is: How should you ease yourself into IF to ensure you achieve your goals?

Chapter 3:
Transitioning into Intermittent Fasting

While all of us would wish this were true, lifestyle changes cannot be adopted at the drop of a hat. The only exception to this is when you're already used to making a raft of changes in your life. For the majority of us though, the minute our brains detect a major shift in behavior, they jump in and seek to preserve the way things are.

This is just how the brain is and there's no reasoning with it. Instead, you should look to be smarter when incorporating change in your life. This chapter is going to show you how to transition into an IF lifestyle that you can stick to. A lot of it is about simplifying the things you need to do. Remember: Simplicity is at the core of success when it comes to dieting!

Transition Programs

In the previous chapter, you learned all about the different IF protocols and how they differ from one another. As you read them you might have already identified the ones which are the most suitable for you to implement in your life. Whatever your chosen protocol is, I still recommend that you follow the week by week plan outlined in the sections below.

This will guarantee that you will stick to IF and leave zero room to sabotage yourself. Even if you are an experienced dieter, sticking to this timeline will help you make better progress over the long run since the changes will be incremental and your body and mind will be able to process the changes better.

Week Zero

The real work begins before you even begin. Don't think of this work as being extremely onerous. The fact is that you'll already have almost everything you need to begin. This week is all about running through checklists and making sure you have all the things you need. This involves making sure you have a meal prep plan, have stocked your kitchen with all the food you need and have made sure you have all the kitchen utensils and miscellaneous things you need to get started.

The second half of this chapter deals will all things meal prep so make sure you read through it thoroughly. A lot of it will seem like common sense but it pays to cover all bases. After all, the smallest thing has the potential to derail your progress and you don't want that to happen.

Once you've gone through all the tasks in the meal prep section, it's time to move onto the first week. This is where you'll be starting your IF protocol for real!

Week One

The first week is marked by the start of the Crescendo method of intermittent fasting. As outlined in the previous chapter, in this method you'll be implementing an intermittent fast for two days of the week and will be eating normally for the rest of it. The aim is to gauge your body's reactions to the new diet regime and monitor yourself for any symptoms that indicate you're not handling things well.

Some of the symptoms to watch out for are:

- Excessive weakness on fasting days - You can expect lower energy levels on the days you fast as your body adjusts but usually, these symptoms will go away by the next day.

- Excessive hunger - Again, some levels of hunger will be present as you enter your fasting window or towards the end of it. If you feel stressed out or cannot concentrate on your tasks, this is a problem. Break your fast and eat something immediately.

- Physical symptoms - Monitor yourself for any menstrual changes and for symptoms like physical pain or bloating etc. All of these could indicate larger issues and you should consult your doctor immediately.

- Dehydration - When you start restricting calories, your body begins to let go of any excess water it holds. If you don't replenish this water you're likely to get dehydrated. Symptoms of this include headaches, dizziness and stress. The ideal amount of water for women to consume on a daily basis is 11.5 cups.

- Exercise fatigue - You'll be starting your chosen exercise regime this week. Start slow and monitor yourself for symptoms of overtraining and excessive fatigue. I'll talk all about exercise in a later chapter so make sure you review the material there.

For most people, the first week will seem pretty uneventful. In terms of results, it's far too soon to be expecting anything. The biggest event that will happen is your body will start letting go of any excess water it has stored. Water storage happens thanks to consuming high levels of carbs throughout the day.

As you implement a fasting window, your body will realize it doesn't need as much water as it has and you'll consequently feel the urge to pee with greater frequency. I don't mean to say you'll be visiting the toilet every five minutes. It's just that you should not be alarmed by what's happening.

As mentioned earlier, you should monitor yourself for symptoms of dehydration since this is a common occurrence when excess water is being shed. Track your water consumption by buying a water bottle and drinking regularly from it. Remember that exercise causes water loss as well and you should be drinking above the daily recommended amount that was mentioned previously.

With regards to the IF days themselves, you might be wondering what an ideal partition time is? As I mentioned in the previous chapter, a 16/8 fasting/feeding window is the best. Practically, this is how it would work. Let's assume your schedule looks something like the one below:

Non-fasting day

8:30PM - Dinner ends and fasting window begins
10PM - Bed
Overnight transition into fasting day
6AM - Wake Up
7AM - Usual breakfast time. Skip on fasting day
12:30PM - Lunch. Breakfast of 16 hours with this meal
8:30PM - Last meal before eight-hour feeding window closes

Overnight transition into a normal day

6AM- Wake Up
7AM - Breakfast

The biggest qualm most people will have is that they will be skipping breakfast on fasting days. I'll address this in the chapter on the myths and tips on implementing IF. For now, understand that breakfast is not the most important meal of the day as the popular myth has you believe.

In fact, no single meal is the most important one of the day. It's all about calories in versus out as you've learned already.

Week Two

Assuming everything was fine in Week One, it's time to move into the second week. Here you'll be adding at least one additional day of IF to your regime. Towards the end of the week, if you feel as if you've adjusted well enough, feel free to add an additional day.

The second week is when your body will adjust itself to the new regime and you won't face additional difficulties adding an extra day of fasting. A great thing to do is to look to add a consecutive fasting day. For example, you'll begin by having three fasting days this week. Let's say these days are Sunday, Tuesday and Thursday.

Add another fasting day on Friday or Wednesday and see how it goes. By adding Wednesday into your protocol, you'll be fasting on three consecutive days, so this might be too big a step for most people. Friday works better from a timing perspective but keep your social engagements in mind and see if you can make it work.

If an additional day (beyond three days) feels excessive at this point, don't worry. This is normal for a lot of people since it can be hard to give up eating breakfast. You can fully expect your stomach to make noises and rumble in the mornings. The key is to apply some awareness in such moments and ask yourself whether you're actually hungry or if you are craving breakfast.

One creative way to solve this issue is to have breakfast food during your first meal. Breakfast food is pretty delicious and there's no need to deprive yourself of it just because you're skipping the meal itself.

As always watch out for any physical symptoms that indicate your body is not adjusting well. By this point, you should not be feeling any diet-related dizziness. If you do feel dizzy, check to see whether you're eating enough food to keep up with the calories you're burning while exercising. The easiest way to do this is to monitor your weight.

If you're losing more than one pound of body weight per week you're probably eating too little. If you see your weight fluctuate more than this on a daily basis, reduce the intensity of your workouts for a week and eat more food. The other thing you can track is your mental state.

Feelings of excessive stress, irritability and an inability to concentrate are signs of your body not receiving enough calories to fuel itself. In addition, watch out for any signs of bloating or abdominal cramps. Bloating occurs when your body doesn't receive enough food and this causes a buildup of gas. Any signs of discomfort in your stomach is an indication that something isn't right and you should immediately tone down the level of change and go back to the previous level where everything was fine.

As this week ends you'll need to plan ahead for the next one. At this point, if you've successfully added an additional day of IF, you should take things up a notch by moving onto a modified 16/8 method as outlined in the previous chapter. If not, follow the Crescendo method next week as well and look to adding another day of IF.

If you're taking things up a level, then you'll need to plan your week ahead and set aside windows for exercise. Since the modified 16/8 adopts the exercise principles of Leangains, your workouts are going to go up a level in terms of intensity. Refer to the chapter on exercise later in this book and decide on which method of exercise works best for you.

It isn't necessary for you to hit the gym although this is ideal. The point is that while walking as a form of exercise was fine until this point, it's not going to cut it anymore. You need to move and break a sweat to a higher degree. Everyone has a different level they need to hit so it is essential that you follow the guidelines in the chapter on exercise to determine where you stand.

Week Three

This week is where you'll either make a bigger change or you'll continue adding more days to the Crescendo method. Either way, you will feel some changes within yourself. It might be greater levels of energy or it might be a different relationship with food. If you're aligning your fasting windows to skip breakfast, your body will get used to it by now and those breakfast pangs will disappear.

This week will be difficult because of the higher intensity of your workouts. Monitor yourself for symptoms of excessive training and a lack of adequate levels of food intake. These symptoms were outlined previously when talking about Week Two. You might be wondering why you need to take things up a notch? Why not stick to the Crescendo method throughout?

The reason is that your body will adjust to the method quite quickly and you won't really see the full benefits of IF. Remember, with the Crescendo method you're actually fasting for a lesser period of time than you are not. If you fast for four days of the week, you might as well implement the modified 16/8.

The biggest complaint usually has to do with the higher intensity of exercise that is required. Remember, the intensity is relative. You don't need to start exercising like an athlete. You simply need to take things to a higher level. The thing about exercise, as you'll learn in a later chapter, is that your body will get used to it pretty soon. In order to make progress, you need to change things up every once in a while and increase your intensity.

This doesn't mean you need to keep increasing it indefinitely. At some point, you'll attain the physique you'll be satisfied with and that is when you can maintain your regime.

However, until you reach that point, you should look to incrementally take things up a notch. You'll learn how to do this so don't worry about this right now.

Week three is when you'll continue monitoring yourself. If you've made it this far, your body has presumably adjusted to IF and you shouldn't be seeing any major symptoms. By the end of the week, if you find the modified 16/8 working for you, this is great! Stick with it and continue doing what you're doing.

If you find it stressful, shift back to the Crescendo method for the following week and look at implementing IF for four days of the week. This means you'll have a couple of days of IF back to back at the very least. At any time during week three if you feel that the rate of change is too high, go back to what was working in the previous week.

There's no need to be pedantic about the changes you're making. Always remember to keep things as comfortable as possible for you but at the same time, you want to be a little uncomfortable. It takes some time to find this ideal spot so don't worry about making changes that are too big or are too small to rate. Trust that you'll eventually find the sweet spot.

Week Four

By the end of this week, you'll have been intermittently fasting for a month! There's still this week to get through though. If you were on the Crescendo method at the end of last week, adopt the modified 16/8 approach. The only exception is if you dialed things down to the Crescendo method after the modified 16/8 was too much for you.

Either way, by the end of this week, try to see if the modified 16/8 works for you. The aim is to be on this protocol by the end of the month. If you can't make this timeline, there's no reason to worry. Simply stick with what's working for you. While the modified 16/8 will bring you massive results, it's not as if you won't see progress with the Crescendo method.

Monitor your diet and weight levels. This goes for your fluid levels as well. Remember, if you're losing more than one pound per week or if you've lost more than this amount over the month, you're not eating enough.

Beyond Week Four

As you move on with IF, you should consider adopting the Leangains approach. This means you'll have to count calories and track macros. If this seems like too much for you then there's no need for you to do it. However, I would encourage you to try it out at least once.

You might find it easier than you thought. Either way, seek to make progress with your exercise and look to become as active as you can be. Exercise by itself is not going to help you lose weight but it will help you build muscle which will replace the fat in your body.

After a month, you will have a good idea of how your body reacts to IF and you'll be able to figure out what works and what doesn't. So trust your judgment and listen to what your body is telling you.

Let us now look at how you can make things easier for yourself when you decide to implement IF. Let's go back all the way to week zero and look at prepping!

IF Prep

Prepping for IF is really all about aligning the various things in your life so as to make adopting IF as easy as possible. This involves meal prep, exercise prep and meal timing. Let's begin by looking at meal prep first.

Meal Prep

Meal prep begins with sorting out your grocery list. The best way to begin IF is to stock your kitchen with staple whole foods that you can create meals from. The next chapter will give you recipes you can create from these. The idea is to have a base of ingredients which will minimize your need to buy a bunch of different things when you shop.

Here's what you need to buy:

- Your choice of grain
  - ○ Choice of rice
  - ○ Whole wheat pasta
  - ○ Quinoa
  - ○ Wheat-based noodles or grains
- Oil
  - ○ Coconut
  - ○ Extra virgin olive oil
  - ○ Rice bran oil
- Protein
  - ○ Meat or animal-based
  - ○ Eggs
  - ○ Tofu and Tempeh if you're vegan
- Vegetables
  - ○ Leafy greens
  - ○ Starchy veggies
    - ■ Potatoes
    - ■ Carrots
  - ○ Onions
  - ○ Tomatoes
- Your choice of fruits
- Dairy
  - ○ Choice of milk
  - ○ Cheese
- Spices
  - ○ Ethnic spice mixes such as five spice or Indian masala powders

- O Paprika
- O Turmeric
- O Cumin
- O Rosemary
- O Oregano
- O Basil
- O Thyme
- O Salt
- O Pepper (black)
- Tomato puree
- Garlic and ginger (paste or whole)
- Whole oats
- Assorted nuts and seeds
- Peanut butter (or any seed butter)
- Cocoa powder or syrup (to make smoothies)
- Ice
- Yogurt
  - O Preferably Greek yogurt. If you don't like yogurt, milk of your choice works

Your first shopping trip is going to take a bit longer than the others if you don't have these items stocked to begin with. The biggest obstacle to meal prep is the lack of interest in some people when it comes to cooking. I get it. Standing in the kitchen waiting for your meals to cook can be exhausting and you have other stuff to get done.

Here's the easy way to get cooking.

Cooking Techniques

The first thing to understand is that not all food cooks the same way or tastes the same once cooked. I know this sounds obvious but you'll be surprised at how many people cook chicken the way they cook fish. Here are a few handy tips to remember:

- Chicken needs a lot of spices to taste good and should be cooked all the way through. Chicken thighs have more fat on them and are tastier. Chicken breasts have no fat on them and are high in protein but need assistance from herbs and sauces to taste good. Thighs don't need as much but they certainly need help.

- Beef and lamb are best left undercooked. You might as well chew on leather than chew a well-done piece of steak or lamb. In most cases, you need a simple sauce and salt and pepper with veggies on the side to make a meal.

- Fish cooks very quickly and should be cooked well to avoid poisoning. Be very careful with what else you handle when touching raw fish. You are not a sushi master so don't experiment with raw fish at the start.

- Substitute smoothies and milkshakes for solid food as breakfast. Throw fruits and veggies along with cocoa powder or peanut butter. Add more of this if you wish to override any other taste.

- If you can stomach it, eat eggs raw. This saves cooking time and you'll eat the highest amount of protein. Blend them into your smoothies to skip the slimy texture.
- Snack healthy by having a smoothie or a handful of nuts.
- Cook meals in batches and reheat them prior to meals.
- You can make an easy sauce by using tomato puree, garlic, salt, and pepper. Add spices or herbs to get it to taste different.
- You can make easy soups by boiling veggies and blending them.

Following these tips will make your life in the kitchen a lot easier. In addition to this, look to bake as much of your food as possible. Baking requires initial prep and then you let the oven do its thing. Cooking on a skillet or even a crockpot requires you to be present. If you have a smart oven, your task is even easier!

The best part about the oven is that you can cook pretty much anything in there. Cook times on a skillet vary on the type of food. Besides, not all food cooks evenly. Try frying chicken breast versus fish on a skillet and you'll know what I'm on about. Besides, with an oven, you're guaranteed an even cook whereas this is not the case with a skillet.

Crockpots and slow cookers are also of great help but you need to make sure you don't burn your food. Speaking of cookware, let's take a look at the utensils and appliances you'll need at a minimum.

Appliances and Utensils

Here's a simple list to help you get started. Remember, this is just a basic list. You can add whatever you want to this list as per your choice.

- Oven
- Skillet
- Crockpot/slow cooker
- Food processor (this does many more things than a blender does so it's a good investment)
- Knives
- Spoons
- Forks
- Bowls/plates
- Tongs
- Spatulas
- Food storage containers
- Baking dish
- Baking sheets
- Sieve/Strainer
- Glasses/cups

That's pretty much it!

Figure Out Your Schedule

The point of preparing meals is to minimize your time in the kitchen. Obviously, if you're someone who loves to cook and who loves the freshest food possible, you won't have any issues. However, a lot of people have other things going on and they need to find a way to utilize their time in the kitchen in the most efficient way possible.

There are two ways of approaching cooking your meals. The first is to cook them in large batches. Generally speaking, you should cook your meals for a maximum of three days and not more than this. According to USDA storage guidelines, most food tends to get spoiled or lose its nutritional value beyond this point (Morin, 2019).

Thus, you'll be cooking two days per week at a minimum. To determine what to cook, you need to design your meals first. The recipes and meal plan in the next chapter will reduce the burden for you. When designing your own meals try to keep the base of them as similar as possible.

For example, you could cook a large batch of rice and then vary things by eating it with chicken during the day and fish at night. Alternatively, you could fry the rice with an egg and eat it with a salad on the side. Another way to approach batch cooking is to bake protein ahead of time and then mix it with salad or rice. You can prep your salad ingredients ahead of time and simply mix everything together when the time comes to eat it.

The second method of approaching meal prep is to prepare batches of ingredients instead of the finished product. You can measure appropriate portions of ingredients and cut them or prep them as needed and cook them together prior to having your meal. This takes more time, obviously but the advantage here is that your meals will be fresh and tasty.

One problem with batch cooking your meals is that you'll lose some of the original texture and every subsequent meal will be less tasty than the previous one. Some people don't mind this and view food as a means of nutrition while some need tasty meals to be satisfied.

You'll need to tailor your approach based on how you feel about all this obviously.

Cheat Meals

A cheat meal is a great way to interrupt any boredom in your meal plan. This is most applicable to those who cook their food in batches. It can get boring to eat the same stuff over and over and you might find that you don't have the patience or desire to stand in the kitchen for long hours.

In such cases, feel free to have something of your choice during one of your meals. For example, Martin Berkhan, the founder of Leangains is particularly famous for his 'demolishing' of entire cheesecakes during the holiday season. Yes, I'm talking about eating an entire cheesecake, not just a slice.

I'm not advocating you go as wild as him but feel free to have a pizza or some junk food you're craving once a week. You don't need to develop an adversarial relationship with food. While processed food is not good for our bodies, it isn't going to cause harm when ingested in small doses. After all, our bodies are a lot more resilient than we think.

Don't overdo it though. Watch out for your desire to turn a cheat meal into a cheat day which morphs into a cheat week. The best time to have a cheat meal is when you're breaking your fast. Most people tend to sleep during their fasting periods so it's not ideal to eat empty calories or bad calories at this time since your body is going to burn less of it.

Timing your cheat meal to the start of the feeding window ensures you will burn all of it since your body is hungry at this point in time.

All in all, meal prep requires a little advance planning and with a little attention, you'll end up incorporating IF into your lifestyle without a hitch.

Chapter 4:
Tasty Recipes and Meal Plan

This chapter is going to simplify cooking further for you by giving you easy recipes you can cook. They require ingredients that are easily found and you don't need to break the bank buying them. Let's begin by looking at a few breakfast recipes.

Breakfast

Even if you choose to skip breakfast, you can eat them at any point during the day. Breakfast food is almost always delicious, so don't be afraid to indulge in them.

One Bowl Turmeric Porridge

For best results, use steel-cut oats. Prepping steel cut oats takes some time due to the fact that you need to soak them overnight for at least six hours. You can use instant oats as well if that's what you prefer. You can cook batches of this and reheat it whenever you wish to eat it. Additionally, you can add peanut butter to the mix to give it a creamier texture.

Serves: Two

Nutrition:

- Total Calories - 430
- Protein - 13
- Carbs - 75

- Fat - 5

Ingredients:

- One cup steel cut oats/ instant oats
- 1.5 cups water
- 1.5 tsp turmeric powder
- ¼ tsp ginger, ground
- ¼ tsp cinnamon powder
- Pinch of pepper
- ½ cup milk
- 2 tbsp maple syrup/Stevia

Steps:

1. If you're using steel-cut oats, soak overnight for at least six hours. Make sure water covers the oats completely.
2. Once soaked, add oats, milk, and water to a saucepan and simmer over low heat. Keep cooking until oats turn soft or have absorbed all the water. If oats stick to the bottom of the pan, add more water. Remove from heat.
3. Add turmeric, ginger, cinnamon, and pepper to the oats and stir well.
4. Serve hot!

Creamy Turmeric Smoothie

Serves: One

Nutrition:

- Total Calories - 300

- Protein - 4
- Carbs - 40
- Fat - 12

Ingredients:

- One cup banana, preferably frozen, sliced
- One cup milk
- ½ tsp turmeric powder, ground
- 1 tbsp ginger, minced
- Pinch of pepper and cinnamon powder

Steps:

1. Add all ingredients to a blender and blitz together until everything is mixed well.
2. Pour into a glass and enjoy!

Green Smoothie With Avocado

This smoothie feels heavier on the stomach and also makes for a great meal replacement shake. Smaller quantities of it make a great snack to tide you over between meal times.

Serves: Two

Nutrition:

- Total Calories - 150
- Protein - 7
- Carbs - 18
- Fat - 5

Ingredients:

- One large banana, preferably frozen, sliced
- ½ medium avocado, pitted and sliced
- One scoop protein powder (see supplements chapter)
- Large handful of kale or greens of your choice
- One cup milk

Steps:

1. Add all ingredients to a blender and blitz till creamy and smooth. Some might find the combination of greens and bananas not sweet enough. You can add a little maple syrup or cocoa powder to sweeten the smoothie up a bit.
2. Pour into a glass and enjoy!

Breakfast Protein Bars

These protein bars are great for breaking your fast and are a great choice as a snack as well. Best of all, you can make them ahead of time. Even better, you don't need to bake them. Simply chill them in your fridge and you're good to go!

Serves: Nine bars

Nutrition:

- Total Calories - 200
- Protein - 11
- Carbs - 13
- Fat - 10

Ingredients:

- ⅓ cup amaranth
- 3 tbsp protein powder (see supplements chapter for more)
- 2 tbsp maple syrup or stevia
- One cup creamy peanut butter
- 3 tbsp melted dark chocolate (not milk chocolate since this contains a ton of sugar)

Steps:

1. The first step to take is to 'pop' the amaranth. This is done by heating a large pot to a suitable level. Add a few drops of water to the pot. If you see it boil as soon as it hits the surface, begin adding amaranth and cover the pot. Shake it overheat until you hear the seeds popping inside. This should take around ten seconds or so.
2. Transfer to a cup and let it cool.
3. Add peanut butter, protein powder and maple syrup until you have a dough-like texture.
4. Transfer this mixture to a baking dish and press to level.
5. Transfer the baking dish to your freezer for around twenty minutes.
6. Remove from freezer and cut into nine bars. Drizzle melted chocolate on top and enjoy!
7. Alternatively, drizzle the chocolate and place it in your fridge or freezer to consume later.

Meal Recipes

These easy recipes are healthy and can be made in batches for you to reheat easily. Some of them require slightly complex cooking techniques but over time, you'll find it easy to make them.

Salmon and Broccoli Lunch Bowl

Despite the word lunch in the name you can eat this whenever you please.

Serves: Four

Nutrition:

- Total Calories - 500
- Protein - 35
- Carbs - 70
- Fat - 7

Ingredients:

- One cup rice
- One tbsp cornstarch
- ¼ cup soy sauce
- Three cloves garlic
- One tbsp ginger
- Four 5oz Salmon fillets
- Three cups broccoli florets

Steps:

1. Preheat your oven to 400F.
2. Cook rice in a saucepan by adding around two cups of water. Alternatively, you can use a rice cooker for this. Set aside.
3. Stir cornstarch and ¼ cup water together. In a saucepan, add soy sauce, garlic, ginger, and the cornstarch mix. Add one cup of water. Mix well together and remove from heat once thick Set aside to cool.
4. On a baking dish, line the salmon fillets and drizzle the sauce from the previous step on top.
5. Bake until the fillets flake. This should take around 15 minutes or so.
6. Meanwhile, boil the broccoli florets for five minutes until soft.
7. Place the rice in a bowl along with salmon and broccoli and serve hot!

BBQ Chicken Salad/Sandwich

The primary dish here is a salad but you can turn this into a sandwich by placing the ingredients between two slices of bread.

Serves: Four

Nutrition:

- Total Calories - 400
- Protein - 30

- Carbs - 25
- Fat - 20

Ingredients:

- One tbsp extra virgin olive oil
- 2 chicken breasts, boneless, skinned
- Salt and pepper to taste
- Six cups lettuce, chopped
- One tomato, diced
- ¾ cup corn kernels
- ¾ cup cooked black beans (canned are fine)
- ¼ cup onions, diced
- One cup shredded cheese (cheddar is fine)
- ¼ cup ranch dressing
- ¼ cup BBQ sauce

Steps:

1. Preheat your own to 375F.
2. On a baking sheet, line the chicken breast and drizzle them with olive oil. Cook until well done. This should take around 15-20 minutes.
3. Dice them into smaller pieces.
4. Assemble the salad in a bowl by placing lettuce, beans, tomato, onion, corn, and cheese. Place the cooked chicken on top and drizzle BBQ sauce and ranch dressing on top.

You can substitute a blend of cheeses if cheddar is not your preferred choice.

Burrito Bowl

Who doesn't love a good burrito! Like with the previous recipe, you can turn this bowl into a burrito by adding the ingredients to a tortilla and wrapping them up.

Serves: Six

Nutrition:
- Total Calories - 380
- Protein - 13
- Carbs - 59
- Fat - 10

Ingredients:
- One cup rice
- One cup salsa. You can use store-bought. Alternatively, chop 3/4 cup tomato and mix with one jalapeno pepper with ¼ small onion, chopped.
- Three cups lettuce, chopped
- One can corn, drained
- One can cooked black beans, drained
- Two tomatoes, diced
- One avocado, pitted and diced
- Two tbsp cilantro, chopped
- One cup sour cream
- One clove garlic
- One tsp lime juice
- Salt to taste

Steps:

1. Combine the last four ingredients in a bowl and mix together. Set aside.
2. Cook rice in a cooker or in a saucepan with two cups of water.
3. In a bowl, assemble rice with all other ingredients. Toss together to ensure they mix well.
4. Enjoy!

This recipe doesn't reheat very well and will lose its texture. If you're making this as a batch, it's best to consume it over two days at the most.

Steak Fajita

Here's another recipe you can have with a tortilla/bread or as a salad. As written, this recipe will result in a salad.

Serves: Six

Nutrition:

- Total Calories - 590
- Protein - 38
- Carbs - 15
- Fat - 42

Ingredients:

- Two tbsp extra virgin olive oil
- One medium onion, sliced
- Three bell peppers, sliced. Preferably of different color

- Eight cups lettuce, chopped
- One avocado, pitted and sliced

Dressing ingredients

- ½ cup sour cream
- One cup cilantro, chopped
- Two tbsp mayonnaise
- Two cloves garlic
- One tbsp lime juice
- ¼ cup extra virgin olive oil
- Salt to taste

Steak Rub

- Two lbs lean steak, cut of your choice
- ¼ cup extra virgin olive oil
- Two cloves garlic, minced
- One tbsp lime juice
- One tsp red paprika powder
- One tsp cumin powder
- One tsp oregano, powdered or dried
- ½ tsp onion powder
- Salt and pepper to taste

Steps:

1. Add all ingredients of the dressing in a food processor, except for the oil. As you pulse them together steadily add oil until it combines and achieves your desired consistency. Set aside.

2. Prepare the marinade for the steak by combining all the ingredients together (except for the meat). Stir in a bowl together and place the steak into this mix. Alternatively, you can combine everything into a plastic resealable bag and marinate it. Make sure you marinate the steak for at least 30 minutes.

3. While marinating, prepare the vegetables. Add oil to pan along with the onion. Caramelize the onions over low heat. This takes around ten minutes. Look for them to become lightly browned.

4. Add bell peppers and cook until tender. Set aside in a separate bowl.

5. Remove steak from marinade and cook over medium heat. Cook to your desired level and remove from heat.

6. Cut the steak into smaller pieces against the grain.

7. In a bowl, place the lettuce and arrange the onion and bell pepper mix. Place the avocado on top of this and top it with the steak.

8. Pour the dressing from the first step over it all and enjoy!

As you can imagine, this dish doesn't reheat very well. If you wish to cook it as a batch, you can make the dressing and the salad portion in advance. It's best to cook the steak fresh. You can marinate large quantities of it overnight prior to cooking individual portions.

Roasted Shrimp Sandwich

This filling sandwich is really taken to another level thanks to the sauce within it.

Serves: Four

Nutrition:
- Total Calories - 250
- Protein - 20
- Carbs - 30
- Fat - 5

Ingredients:
- One pound shrimp, shelled and deveined
- One tsp garlic powder
- ½ tsp paprika powder
- Salt and pepper to taste
- Lettuce for filling
- ½ avocado, pitted and sliced for filling

Dressing ingredients
- Three chipotle peppers in adobo sauce, store-bought
- One avocado, pitted and chopped
- ¼ cup mayonnaise
- ¼ cup regular or Greek yogurt (Greek yogurt will increase the protein content)
- One tbsp lime juice
- Salt to taste

Steps:

1. Preheat your oven to 400F.
2. Combine all the ingredients of the dressing in a food processor and pulse until combined together. If you want a thicker sauce you can add more yogurt.
3. Combine the rest of the ingredients in a bowl together. Make sure the shrimp is well coated with the spices.
4. Place shrimp on a baking dish and cook in the oven for around seven minutes or until well done.
5. You can serve as a sandwich on a baguette or between two slices of bread. Spread some of the dressing on each slice, place lettuce and avocado along with shrimp. Enjoy!

Chicken and Pesto Sandwich

This twist on an Italian classic will leave you hungry for more!

Serves: Four

Nutrition:

- Total Calories - 310
- Protein - 30
- Carbs - 40
- Fat - 8

Ingredients:

- Two cups cooked chicken breast, shredded
- ¼ cup Greek yogurt or regular yogurt

- Two tomatoes, sliced
- Eight oz mozzarella, sliced

Pesto ingredients

- One cup basil leaves
- Three cloves garlic
- Three tbsp pine nuts
- ⅓ cup Parmesan cheese, grated
- ⅓ cup extra virgin olive oil
- Salt and pepper to taste

Steps:

1. Combine all ingredients for the pesto in a food processor, except for the oil, and pulse. While pulsing add the oil slowly as the mixture gains consistency. Set aside.
2. In a bowl combine the rest of the ingredients together along with the pesto from the previous step and add salt and pepper to taste.
3. Serve on bread as a sandwich!

In case you're wondering how to cook the chicken, you can chop it into small pieces and saute it in a pan with salt and pepper until it's well cooked. Alternatively, you can bake the breasts in the oven until well done. Make sure you drizzle them with olive oil and sprinkle them with salt and pepper prior to baking.

Desserts

You need to eat healthy sure but this doesn't mean you should not indulge your sweet tooth. Desserts don't equal sugar and these healthy, easy to make desserts can be had as a sweet end to your feeding window or as a snack somewhere in between.

Berry Compote

Technically this is a topping but you can use this to turn almost anything into a dessert. Top your yogurt or a pancake mix with this compote for an instant dessert!

Serves: Six

Nutrition:
- Total Calories - 27
- Protein - 1
- Carbs - 6
- Fat - negligible

Ingredients:
- Three cups frozen or fresh berries (strawberries, raspberries, cherries etc)
- Three tbsp orange juice
- ¼ tsp ginger, ground
- ¼ tsp cinnamon

Steps:
1. In a saucepan, place the fruit and juice and gently bring to medium heat.
2. Once it bubbles, reduce the heat and mash the fruit.

3. Keep stirring and cooking over low heat as the mixture thickens and the fruit combines with the juice better.

4. Remove from heat and add ginger and cinnamon.

5. Transfer to a container and cool it in the fridge.

No-Bake Chocolate Cake Bites

Chocolate is a safe go-to for a lot of dessert lovers. This recipe, like the one before it will satisfy the vegans reading this as well!

Serves: 15 bites

Nutrition:
- Total Calories - 115
- Protein - 4
- Carbs - 17
- Fat - 5

Ingredients:
- One cup dates, pitted
- One cup almond flour
- ⅓ cup coconut flour
- ¼ cup cocoa powder
- Two tsp vanilla extract
- Four tbsp maple syrup/stevia
- One tbsp coconut cream (you can also substitute full-fat milk in here if not vegan)

Steps:

1. Pulse dates in a food processor until they're cut into small bits. Usually a ball forms if the dates are sticky enough. Scoop out and set aside.
2. Add both flours and cocoa powder and blend for half a minute or so.
3. Add the dates, vanilla, maple syrup and coconut cream. Pulse until a dough forms.
4. Scoop out around 1.5 to two tbsp of dough and roll it into balls. Arrange these on a baking tray and place them in the freezer once all of the dough is used up.
5. Freeze for around ten minutes. Enjoy!

You can prepare a glaze for the bites as well by melting dark chocolate. Alternatively, you can mix cocoa powder with butter and coconut oil together and coat the frozen bites with the glaze. Freeze them for another ten minutes so that the glaze hardens.

Peanut Butter Cookies

Peanut butter cookies. Need I say more? Best of all, these don't need any baking whatsoever!

Serves: 12 cookies

Nutrition:

- Total Calories - 170
- Protein - 4

- Carbs - 25
- Fat - 7

Ingredients:

- One cup oats
- ¾ cup dates, pitted
- ½ cup creamy peanut butter
- Salt to taste

Steps:

1. Add oats and salt to a food processor and pulse until fine. Add dates to this and blend for another 40 seconds. Add peanut butter and blend some more until a dough forms.
2. Scoop out two tbsp of dough at a time and form mounds of them. Line them on a baking tray and chill for ten minutes or so.
3. Alternatively, you can enjoy them immediately.

The glaze that you can make for the previous recipe can be used here as well. You can drizzle the glaze over the cookies and freeze the cookies until the glaze hardens.

Spicy Fruit Salad

A perfect salad for summer with a blend of healthy fruits and just enough spice to keep it interesting.

Serves: Six

Nutrition:

- Total Calories - 110
- Protein - 2
- Carbs - 27
- Fat - <1

Ingredients:

- Two mangoes, peeled and cubed
- Four kiwis, peeled and sliced
- One cup strawberries, sliced
- One cup blueberries
- Two tbsp lime juice
- ¼ tsp paprika powder
- One tbsp maple syrup
- Salt to taste

Steps:

1. Add all fruits to a bowl and mix together. Add lime juice and maple syrup and gently toss together.
2. Add salt to taste and sprinkle paprika powder. Make sure you fold it into the salad well.
3. Chill for ten minutes and serve.

You can use any combination of fruit for this salad. As long as the fruits are on the sweeter side they'll go well with the spiciness of the paprika.

Vegan-Friendly Meal Recipes

To satisfy the vegans among us, here are four delicious vegan recipes you can create easily. Being a vegan isn't the easiest thing so these recipes will lighten the burden of figuring out what to eat considerably.

Black Bean and Sweet Potato Chili

This recipe takes around an hour to put together but is oh-so delicious!

Serves: Six

Nutrition:
- Total Calories - 215
- Protein - 7
- Carbs - 50
- Fat - 1

Ingredients:
- One medium onion diced
- One tbsp extra virgin olive oil
- Three sweet potatoes, medium, chopped
- 16oz store-bought salsa
- 15 oz can cooked black beans
- Two cups vegetable stock
- 2 cups water
- One tbsp paprika powder
- Two tsp cumin powder
- Salt to taste

Steps:

1. In a large pot, add oil and onion and cook until translucent. Add salt and pepper to taste.
2. Add sweet potato along with paprika powder and cumin to the mix.
3. Add salsa, water and vegetable stock.
4. Bring to a boil on medium heat and simmer. Add black beans and cover. Cook for another 30 minutes or so.
5. You can make the soup thicker by mashing the sweet potato with a spoon or fork.
6. Let the mixture rest for a while before serving.

You can make this in batches and it stores well in the fridge for up to three days.

Easy Lentil Soup

Lentils are a great vegan source of protein. This soup will fill you up thanks to it being full of fiber.

Serves: Four

Nutrition:

- Total Calories - 370
- Protein - 19
- Carbs - 69
- Fat - 2

Ingredients:

- Two cloves garlic, minced

- Two tbsp coconut or extra virgin olive oil
- Two small onions, diced
- Four large carrots, skinned and sliced
- Four celery stalks (optional)
- Salt and pepper to taste
- Three cups baby potatoes, chopped
- Four cups vegetable stock
- Handful of rosemary and thyme
- One cup uncooked green lentils (rinsed and drained)
- Two cups chopped kale

Steps:

1. Heat a large pot over medium heat. Add oil, garlic, onion, carrots and celery. Add salt and pepper and stir together.
2. Add potatoes and cook together for a couple minutes more.
3. Add veggie stock, rosemary and thyme and increase heat as the mixture simmers. Add lentils and stir. Keep cooking until potatoes and lentils are tender.
4. Add greens and cook until they wilt.
5. Pour into cups and enjoy as a soup.

Alternatively, you could also have this with rice as a curry. Garnish with some fresh coriander leaves for an even better taste!

Vegan Minestrone

Serves: Six

Nutrition:

- Total Calories - 130
- Protein - 10
- Carbs -18
- Fat - 2

Ingredients:

- Two tbsp extra virgin olive oil
- ½ medium onion diced
- Three cloves garlic, minced
- Two large carrots, peeled and sliced
- 1.5 cups green beans, chopped
- One small zucchini, sliced
- 15 oz can roasted tomatoes
- Six cups vegetable stock
- Two tsp basil, dried
- Two tsp oregano, dried
- One tbsp sugar to taste
- 15 oz can cooked chickpeas
- Two cups pasta noodles
- One cup spinach or kale

Steps:

1. In a large pot over medium heat, add oil, onion and garlic. Stir until translucent.

2. Add carrots, green beans and salt and pepper. Cook for four minutes or so until the vegetables have softened.

3. Add zucchini, tomatoes, vegetable stock, basil, oregano, sugar and chickpeas. Stir together well.

4. Increase heat and bring the soup to a simmer. Add pasta and stir together. Cook for another ten minutes making sure that the soup simmers and doesn't boil.

5. Add kale and cook until it wilts. Remove from heat and serve in bowls!

7 Day Meal Plan

You can create a simple meal plan using all of these recipes. If cooking isn't your thing, simply follow the meal plan below to make things easy on yourself.

Day #	First Meal	Second Meal	Third Meal
1	Creamy turmeric smoothie + breakfast protein bars	Black bean and sweet potato chili	Roast shrimp sandwich+peanut butter cookies
2	BBQ chicken salad	Roast shrimp sandwich	Black bean and sweet potato chili + no-bake chocolate cake bites

3	Breakfast porridge with berry compote	Chicken pesto sandwich	Salmon and rice bowl
4	Creamy turmeric smoothie	Burrito bowl + peanut butter cookies	Green smoothie with avocado + no-bake chocolate cake bites
5	Burrito bowl + no-bake chocolate cake bites	Breakfast porridge with berry compote	Steak fajita+peanut butter cookies
6	Green smoothie with avocado	Salmon and rice bowl	Steak fajita
7	Breakfast protein bars with porridge	Vegan minestrone	Burrito bowl

Chapter 5:
Exercise Basics

Exercise is a tough topic for most to get their heads around since there is a lot of misinformation floating around with regards to it. A lot of people think they need special forms of exercise or special programs in order to unlock some special secret to fat loss.

As you'll learn in this chapter, the primary goal of exercise is not to burn fat but to increase strength. Fat loss is taken care of by your nutrition and the amount of muscle you put on. There are many different forms of exercise you can undertake but before looking at all of this, we need to address the sizeable elephant in the room.

Am I Too Old to Exercise?

To be more precise, you might be wondering if 50 is far too old to be exercising with intensity. Your knees and hips might have prompted this question or it might be a purely mental thing. Either way, I'm here to tell you that yes, exercise doesn't come with any numbers attached to it.

Unless you have a debilitating injury of some kind or if your doctor has specifically recommended you stay away from certain forms of exercise, it is perfectly okay for you to undertake all forms of activity. The keyword in all of this is intensity.

How should one determine the ideal level of intensity and how do you know when you're in the sweet spot? To begin with, intensity levels are determined by where you begin. If you've been a couch potato for the last ten years, your ideal intensity level is going to be very different from someone who has been actively exercising for the same amount of time.

As with transitioning into IF, the key is to build your activity levels slowly. Begin by asking yourself what forms of activity do you enjoy? Do you prefer being outside as opposed to in a gym? Or do you prefer the more communal environment a gym offers? One of the benefits of joining fitness programs such as Crossfit is the community that revolves around it and the support you will receive.

A lot of women dismiss gyms thanks to the perceived body shaming or embarrassment that they think occurs. This is not the truth. If anything, the more hardcore the gym you join is, the greater the support you'll receive from the bros who hang out there. This is because almost every powerlifter or bodybuilder started out extremely skinny or overweight before getting into shape.

However, those kinds of gyms are intimidating to join. As long as you can pick an activity you enjoy, make plans to engage in it regularly. If you're the aforementioned couch potato, simply walking briskly for up to an hour in the park every day is a huge achievement.

In addition to planning which activity you enjoy the most, there is one crucial thing you must ensure your workout program has.

Progressive Overload

In powerlifting circles, there is a principle called progressive overload. It's quite simple in theory. A lifter seeks to increase the weight they're lifting in small increments every workout. If they lift 100 lbs today, they look to lift 105 lbs during the next workout or the next time they perform the same exercise. Traditionally, five pounds is the minimum step size when it comes to increasing weight.

The reason this principle works is because it is extremely simple to understand and it works like a charm. Our bodies are extremely resilient. They also happen to be lazy. I don't mean lazy in a Rip Van Winkle sense but more that they seek to become comfortable as soon as possible. If you haven't been exercising you'll find that your body will throw two major hurdles at you.

First, you will find it difficult to get up and go. Once you start moving, your body will squeal in protest at every step. Once it's warmed up, you'll find that the complaints stop and you'll begin to perform the movements well. Over time, you'll find that those movements aren't stressful anymore and that your progress (in terms of performance and muscle growth) will stop.

Progressive overload solves this issue completely. By increasing the weight constantly, it gets your body used to being under stress. In turn, your body adapts to the new regime and begins to treat this as the new normal. Thus, the complaints stopped. Next, by increasing weight, your body is forced to build new muscle to adapt or else it'll simply fall behind. Hence, you make progress in terms of strength since more muscle equals strength.

Does this mean progressive overload will turn you into the Hulk? This is yet another urban legend that a lot of women believe. No amount of weight lifting will ever get you looking like a bodybuilding man, unless you're purposefully aiming for that goal. There's an incalculable amount of evolution built into your curves and biology and a little weightlifting is not going to undo all of that.

You will build muscle but your body will end up looking and feeling stronger. You'll even look more feminine. Don't take my word for it. This is something that Martin Berkhan recommends as well. In his words, if you lift like a man, you'll look like a goddess (Leangains.com, 2020).

Not everyone likes going to the gym however so let's take a look at some forms of exercise you can do outside the gym first.

Forms of Exercise

There are many types of exercise you can undertake. Broadly speaking, these fall into gym oriented or non-gym oriented exercises. There's no denying that it is far easier to build an exercise and strength program around gym-related activities. However, this doesn't mean non-gym related ones aren't beneficial. If anything, your all-round strength will develop better if you exercise outside the gym.

Running/Swimming/Sports etc

All forms of sports are a great way to increase strength. While engaging in any sport, there are two things you need to be aware of. The first is the form you employ when conducting all activities related to the sport. Employing incorrect posture or form is the easiest way to incur an injury and this is going to set you back.

Swimming is one of the best sports you can undertake since it happens to be low impact. Low impact refers to the force your joints have to bear when carrying out the activity. Given that swimming happens in water, your joints bear minimal impact. The downside is that swimming happens to be extremely technical and it's a good idea to hire someone to teach you to swim in case you don't know how.

When starting off with these activities, it pays to start off slow and then slowly build your competence at them. Much like lifters increase the weight per session by five pounds, you can try to carry out the activity or five more minutes per session.

The other thing to keep in mind with regards to such forms of exercise is that your strength will plateau at some point in time. This is because the physical movement you undertake will build your strength up to a certain level and to progress further, you will need to perform greater amounts of that activity or go to the gym and work on increasing your strength.

What I mean is that once you begin swimming well, you will see differences in your arms and back as well as notice that your legs become more toned. However, swimming for half an hour every day for a year is not going to turn you into an Olympic swimmer. To reach anything even mildly resembling an Olympic swimmer's physique, you will need to swim for much more than half an hour or so, not to mention refine your technique.

This is why it pays to go to the gym and work on your strength. Your performance in other areas will increase as well. Lastly, physical activity levels you'll undertake by going to the gym and playing a sport will increase your metabolism and your body will become more efficient at burning whatever you fuel it with.

With this in mind, let's take a look at what you can do in the gym.

Gym Work

Broadly speaking, there are two activities everyone carries out in the gym. They either hit the weights (or train for strength and shape) or perform cardio. Cardio and strength are two ends of a scale and it is physically impossible for human beings to have elite cardio levels and strength levels at the same time (Scott, 2019).

The easiest way of understanding this is to examine Olympic runners. Take a look at the athletes who compete in the 10,000-meter races and you'll see a bunch of people who look malnourished but actually possess extraordinary cardiovascular systems. These athletes look like bags of bones but can run nonstop for half an hour and then still have enough gas in the tank to sprint to the finish.

They don't possess much muscle but have enough of it to power them through whatever task they need to perform. Contrast them with the athletes who take part in the 100-meter race. Those athletes look like a bunch of Greek gods with muscles bulging all over the place. These mountains explode and finish their races in under ten seconds. Running these races is more about power than endurance and thus, they need those large quantities of muscle to push them through.

This doesn't mean to say that a 100-meter Olympic athlete has poor endurance. Far from it. It's just that when compared to other Olympic athletes, they will struggle when switching to longer-lasting disciplines. It doesn't make sense to compare ordinary people to athletes who train every day for close to four years, so comparing them in this way makes more sense.

Ask a 100-meter runner to race in the 10,000-meter race and they'll likely finish last, if they even manage to finish at all. Similarly, a 10,000-meter runner stands no chance of finishing anything but last in a 100-meter sprint. My point is that endurance and power exist on two opposite ends. Your aim should be to find a happy balance between both.

The intensity of your workouts is what determines this. For the average person, working out for strength and then performing some form of cardio for close to ten or fifteen minutes is more than enough to achieve a balance. This is precisely the kind of workout routine that Berkhan recommends as a part of Leangains (Leangains.com, 2020). It isn't just him, every strength training or gym-related program you find will advocate the same thing.

The only difference is in the type of exercise you will be asked to perform. Some programs focus on strength training while others focus on what is called Hypertrophy. Hypertrophy refers to stimulating your muscles to a level where they grow in size. Generally speaking, men benefit a lot more from such workouts than women since men's bodies are better suited for this kind of training.

Your objective should be to train for strength and perform cardio at the end of it. With this in mind, let's take a look at how you can do this.

Workout Programs

The gold standard of strength training workout programs is Starting Strength which was designed by Mark Rippetoe, who is a renowned strength coach. The basis of the program is a series of compound lifts. A compound lift is one which utilizes the largest number of muscles in the body.

An example of a compound lift is a squat. The squat looks pretty straightforward but is actually an extremely complex lift to perform. It involves using the muscles in your legs, core, upper back and chest. Your forearms also get a workout with heavier weight. The other lifts that are a part of Starting Strength are the overhead press, bench press, barbell row, the deadlift and exercises such as pull-ups and dips.

This isn't a book on how to perform those exercises so all I'll say is that you should visit www.strartingstrength.com to understand how the program works and how you should incorporate progressive overload into your lifts. In addition to this, you should take the time to learn the correct form when performing these exercises.

If there's a downside to compound movements, it is that they take a while to learn. You'll need to synchronize large muscle groups in your body and at first, there will be strength imbalances. This will cause you to feel weird and you might end up moving in odd ways.

This is why it's crucial to start with as little weight as possible and to leave your ego at home. The other thing to leave at home is your sense of embarrassment. You will not see a lot of women deadlifting or squatting at the gym and it might be intimidating for you to wade in between the big boys and squat. As I mentioned earlier, once you begin squatting regularly, you'll find those big men will turn into your biggest supporters and will even help you with your lifts. So go ahead and start lifting!

Fasted and Non Fasted

One of the things to keep in mind if or when you move onto the Leangains protocol is to decide whether you wish to train fasted or not fasted. In other words, will you train before you eat anything or during the day when you're in your feeding window. As a beginner to IF, I would never recommend that you train fasted.

This is because you need to have adequate supplementation to preserve muscle when training this way and the slightest mistake will cause you to lose a ton of muscle. Hence, play it safe and workout after you've had a meal or two. Do not work out after your final meal because post-workout nutrition is essential if you wish to make progress.

I'm using the word workout here to imply both gym sessions as well as any sporting activity you choose to undertake. When it comes to fat loss, fasted workouts are the best option. This is because in a fasted state, your body is depleted of glycogen and it has no option but to burn fat for fuel. As long as you can preserve muscle mass, you will drop fat extremely quickly.

Preserving muscle requires experience though, in both the gym as well as with your diet. For starters, you'll need to understand how many supplements you need to take so that your body has an adequate amount of protein to offset any muscle loss. Second, you need to understand the degree of intensity that will work for you when working out. Generally speaking, you should build a good amount of muscle before looking to cut fat.

Follow the modified 16/8 approach for a period of at least six months or so before trying to cut fat. Aside from this, you should also pay attention to your meal times.

Meal Timing

By meal times, I'm not referring to the clock. Instead, I'm referring to how you structure your meals around your activity periods. During your training days, you should aim to eat at least 60% of your calories after your workout. This means your post-workout meal should be the largest of your day and ideally, you'll have a smaller meal after that one.

If you can squeeze in just one meal after your workout, aim to eat 40% of your daily calories in that single meal. It will seem odd for you to divide your meals in this manner but this is what will ensure the majority of your food gets converted into muscle. You don't need to count calories to make sure this happens.

Simply eyeball the amount of food you eat daily and divide it roughly into a 60/40 ratio. During your off days or non-training days, you can spread your calories out more evenly.

When you first transition into IF, you'll be on a two-day cascade program. Aim to workout on your non-fasting days. In week two when you add another day of IF, aim to workout during that day and monitor how you feel. If you can handle it, add another workout during a fasting day and take it slowly from there.

Remember, working out on a fasting day is not the same a working out fasted. You'll be training during the feeding window during your day. This doesn't mean you need to remain comatose during the fasting phase. It's just that you should avoid any strenuous activity during this time.

Cardio Programs

All cardio programs fall into two broad types: Anaerobic and aerobic. The former refers to when you train on an oxygen deficit and the latter is when you have a steady supply of oxygen. Anaerobic exercise is shorter in duration since there's only so long we can function without oxygen.

Strength training and weight lifting take care of the anaerobic portion of cardio pretty well. Once you start lifting heavier weights as the program dictates, you'll train this side of your cardiovascular system. As for the aerobic side, activities such as running and swimming do a great job of training this. Cycling is another activity that you can undertake.

You have two choices when it comes to timing your cardio routine. You can either perform it on alternate days with strength training or you can add a session at the end of it. Alternatively, you can sprinkle in the odd day of sports or cardio training during the week along with performing it at the end of your workout session.

When starting out, I recommend sticking to a small window at the end of your gym session and restricting this time to 15 minutes at the most. The biggest reason for this has to do with resting. Many beginners to exercise underestimate the importance of rest. Real progress isn't made in the gym. It is made when you sleep. This is when your body repairs itself and gets stronger.

You'll find that after a tough workout session, you'll need to sleep for longer periods of time. Your body will adjust over time and you'll find that eight hours will be enough. However, if you were to alternate your cardio and strength days, you'll overwork yourself and are less likely to stick to a regimen.

One of the biggest benefits of a program like Starting Strength is that you'll workout for just three days a week. This is because you'll be performing compound lifts that take a lot out of you. In other words, you have four days of the week left to do whatever you wish instead of being stuck in the gym. Why would you want to reduce this time by performing extended cardio sessions?

Vary your choice of cardio after your workouts. Swim one day, cycle the next, run on the third and so on. The elliptical machine in the gym is also a great choice. If you find yourself exhausted, then feel free to skip cardio altogether. Strength training by itself will bring your cardio capacity up to a good level.

There is one form of cardio that is becoming increasingly popular, especially in Crossfit gyms.

HIIT

HIIT stands for High Intensity Interval Training. This is how it works: You perform an activity extremely fast for a short period, say for half a minute, rest for 20 seconds, and then get back to performing the activity for half a minute again. You repeat this for close to ten to fifteen minutes.

The fact is that HIIT is a great way to lose fat. Perform HIIT while fasted and the fat will practically melt right off. The downside of HIIT is that it can cause muscle loss since you'll have to exert so much more effort. This can be mitigated with proper nutrition (such as eating the majority of your calories after working out or supplementing well when training fasted,) however it isn't recommended for beginners.

You need to have a certain strength level before HIIT makes sense for you to implement. Also, don't think of HIIT as being a workout by itself. Some practitioners choose to portray it this way but HIIT will build your strength to a certain level beyond which you'll need to resort to weights to make progress.

My recommendation is to perform regular, so-called steady-state aerobic cardio, for a period of at least three months before you try HIIT. Once you feel you can handle it at the end of your workouts, look to perform it fasted on non-training days to accelerate your fat loss.

As always, before starting a new exercise regimen, talk to your doctor. They can give you some ideas of how to start to best protect your body and health. This concludes our look at exercise basics. Let's now move onto another important topic, which is supplementation.

Chapter 6:
Supplements

Supplements are not strictly necessary when you begin intermittent fasting. The primary reason for a lot of supplements is to help you with your workouts and to make up for any protein shortfall in your diet. At the start, as long as you're eating enough protein and are eating a fair share of leafy greens, technically speaking you don't need any additional supplements.

However, those on special diets or those who have specific lifestyle choices will suffer from deficiencies. Furthermore, the climate where you live and the seasons can cause imbalances as well.

With this in mind, let's take a look at the supplements you should have at all costs.

The Ones You Need- No Matter What

These supplements are absolutely necessary for you to have. Think of consuming them as making doubly sure you're receiving your appropriate share of micronutrients and other minerals. There's just two of them so it isn't as if this is a huge list.

Multivitamins

Multivitamin tablets are essential even if you aren't following intermittent fasting. As we grow old, micronutrient deficiencies become more pronounced and have more adverse effects than usual (Morin, 2019). The simple fact is that our bodies' resilience decreases as we get older and we need to support them with increasing regularity.

With this in mind, popping a regular dose of multivitamin tablets makes sure you'll receive the appropriate levels of vitamins and minerals. These are especially useful for people who happen to live in areas that experience extreme winters or cold. People in these areas usually suffer from a lack of Vitamin D which is linked to exposure to the sun.

Those who follow a vegan lifestyle are deficient in vitamin B12 thanks to it being found mostly in animal-based products. Multivitamins will help bridge this gap. You don't need any special brand of multivitamin and neither do you need anything tailored for women over 50 or some such arbitrary threshold.

A common misconception that occurs when people begin to ingest multivitamins is that they start losing track of their fluid levels. Here's how it happens. Multivitamin tabs tend to color your pee yellow and this is how most people track their hydration levels. With the increased yellowness, they either assume they're dehydrated or they go the other way and assume they're drinking enough and that all of the yellowness is attributable to the tablets.

So make sure to monitor yourself for other symptoms of dehydration. Even better, get yourself a water bottle and drink from it so that you know you're drinking the right amounts of water every day.

Omega 3

Omega 3 is a type of fatty acid that plays a very important role in a number of bodily functions (Hicks, 2018). Amongst other things, it helps ensure your skin and hair remain shiny and healthy and they also help prevent cancer. This is because Omega 3 is at the forefront of fighting free radicals that cause cancer.

Free radicals are chemicals that can be thought of as being after products of the digestion process. They can be absorbed through the skin as well. For example, chemical-based sunscreen causes free radical damage to the skin, although the levels are extremely low. Either way, free radicals cannot be excreted by the body in their existing shape and need to be flushed by other means.

This is where Omega 3 comes into the picture. The best source of Omega 3 is fish, especially fatty fish like sardines, mackerel, salmon and tuna. Canned fish also contains high levels of

Omega 3. Make it a point to eat a can of fish (or fresh fish as per your choice) to make sure you get a regular dose of this.

If fish is distasteful to you, you can supplement Omega 3 using capsules. Make sure you buy capsules that clearly state they're derived from fish. There are many Omega 3 supplements available that are derived from vegetable sources and these aren't the best. If you're vegan, you'll have to stick to these. It isn't as if plant-sourced Omega 3 is bad. It's just that it isn't the best source.

Omega 3 supplements sometimes also go by the name of cod liver oil. Unless you're vegan, as long as the source of the oil is fish-based, you're good to go.

The Ones You Should Consider

Determining whether you need these supplements or not depends on how you choose to approach intermittent fasting. At the very least, I would recommend storing up on the first one since it can help you meet your protein intake goals pretty easily. As for the others, it depends on your choice of workout and whether you wish to move into fasted training or not.

Protein Powder

A lot of women think protein powder is the same as steroids. This is fortunately untrue. Protein powder is made by dehydrating the strains of protein found in milk. Vegan protein powder is synthesized from plant-based protein sources such as soy. There are two types of non-vegan protein powders you will find (almost every vegan protein powder is soy-based.) These are Casein and whey.

Whey is the more popular form of protein thanks to its fast release qualities. Generally speaking, 32g of whey protein powder contains around 28-30 g of protein. As you can imagine, consuming a few scoops per day will help you hit your protein intake goals pretty easily. You should aim to eat a significant amount of protein via whole food but there's nothing wrong in supplementing in this manner.

It's just that whole food will keep your digestion in check since protein requires additional effort to breakdown. However, if you find that cooking protein is too much of a hassle, or that your schedule is packed, there's nothing wrong in getting the majority of your protein in powder form.

Whey will provide you with an instant boost and is fast-acting. Casein, on the other hand is a slow-acting protein and releases into your bloodstream over time. A lot of bodybuilders consume casein before they go to bed since this ensures their muscles have a steady stream of protein overnight. You don't need to follow this level of discipline.

Generally speaking, whey protein works just fine for everyone. There's no difference in taste between the two types of powders and both of them are available in different flavors.

When choosing a powder, remember that the cheapest isn't always the best. Almost every cheap powder has additional processing carried out on it which results in a higher levels of carbs than a higher quality powder.

Furthermore, you might find that the cheaper powder upsets your digestion and causes bloating. So be wary of them. Brands such an Optimum Nutrition or anything from chains like GNC are a great option. You will sometimes see whey powders branded as whey isolate. This refers to the powder being almost 100% protein. Given that carb levels in all protein powders aren't very high, you don't need to purchase isolates or expect any significant advantage from them.

On average, isolate powder will contain around 2-3g more protein per scoop, which isn't all that much. When it comes to vegans, protein powder is a required supplement. After all, at some point, you're going to get sick of eating tofu or tempeh all the time. One of the deficiencies of the vegan diet is that all high protein sources come with high levels of carbs attached to them.

Lentils, chickpeas etc. are high in carbs and protein. As long as you can burn those carbs via exercise and general activity you'll be fine but not everyone has the time to do this. Protein powder is a great way to make sure you get a concentrated shot of it without having to eat additional carbs.

You can purchase whey and vegan protein powder online or in a store pretty easily.

BCAA

BCAA stands for branched chain amino acids. Think of it this way: Your muscles are made of protein and protein is made of BCAA. All protein powder contains BCAA within it. So why am I mentioning it separately? Well, there's a few differences between regular protein powder and BCAA supplements.

The first is that BCAAs enter the bloodstream directly and thus act faster than protein powder. The second is that BCAAs have far fewer calories, almost zero, compared to protein powder.

This makes them the ideal supplement if you wish to train fasted. There has been some debate about this recently since some research indicates that ingesting BCAA sends a signal to your brain that your fast has been broken and it thus flips into regular mode (Hicks, 2018). However, there is no conclusive research at this point.

As such, you can safely ingest 5-10g BCAA an hour prior to your workout without worrying about breaking your fast. Do not make the mistake of thinking of BCAA as your fasted state protein solution though. While they make for a good pre-workout supplement, they're not a post-workout recovery supplement. Whole food is the best option post-workout, along with a protein shake. Supplements alone should never be your recovery choice.

All in all, until you reach a point where you can consider working out fasted, you really don't need BCAA. You will find BCAA sold in powder as well as capsule form. The powder forms are usually flavored and these have some calories attached to them. So take care and read the nutrition labels carefully before purchasing them.

Creatine

Creatine monohydrate is one of the most thoroughly researched supplements on the market and all in all, the consensus is that it is one of the best supplements for muscle building (Hicks, 2018). Having said that, do you need it?

It isn't as if you're not going to build muscle without creatine so the answer to that is no. If you want it though, feel free to supplement it in your diet. Don't make the mistake of thinking you have to have it.

Fat Burners

Despite the name, fat burners don't burn fat. Think of them as being little espresso shots which get you up and about. If you consume too many of them, you'll likely want to run through a wall so be careful with the dosage. Fat burners are helpful when you train fasted since it can be tough to get up and going first thing in the morning.

There are some kinds of fat burners that your body will get used to and these are usually caffeine-based. A lot of people get the same effect from fat burners as they do from a tall cup of joe so this could be a good option for you.

Other Supplements

There are a number of other supplements available on the market and all of them have appropriately marketable names. You'll find products like mass gainers, fat trimmers, collagen supplements and the 'beast mass muscle blazing XXL isopropylene monohydroxidate' variety of bro science products.

You don't really need them despite what the fitness industry tries to tell you. Remember that human beings got by just fine without supplements for centuries on end. Also, there's a reason they're called 'supplements' and not 'meals.'

Deciding whether you need these products is entirely up to you. In the beginning, you don't need anything other than a multivitamin, Omega 3 and protein powder (if you're vegan or not sure you can eat adequate amounts of protein.) As for the rest, take a call as you gain experience with the IF protocol.

Chapter 7:
Tips and Tricks to Make IF Work

This chapter is all about helping you make your life easier when it comes to implementing intermittent fasting. There are a few pitfalls that a lot of beginners fall into and following these tips will help you avoid them. It isn't just IF tips you'll receive in this chapter, I'll be addressing exercise tips as well.

Let's first take a look at the IF side of things.

Intermittent Fasting Tips

These tips will help you get adjusted to IF quickly once you begin.

Drink Water

I've mentioned this before but it bears repeating. Dehydration is something that can derail you off your path pretty quickly. Your body will let go of any excess water it holds in the beginning and you will see a drop in weight. Don't mistake this for fat loss however, it's just water weight.

Despite this water being considered unnecessary, such a sudden release of fluid can trigger dehydration in some people. The thing to do is to play it safe and prevent it from the start. Purchase a water bottle that has markings on it so you know how much water you're drinking throughout the day.

Aim to drink slightly more than your required intake level and monitor yourself for the symptoms of dehydration I listed earlier in the book. Keep in mind that exercise will result in water loss and you should replenish this water as much as possible. You might be tempted to think that energy drinks will do the job but remember that they contain a lot of sugar and aren't the best option for you.

Stick to good ol' water and you'll be fine.

Plan Ahead

Take some time the night before to plan your day ahead. When will your fasting window end and will you be able to eat a meal at that time? When will you cook and do you need to prep. Prepping is something that tends to catch people out for the most part. This is mostly due to it being a habit they haven't practiced before.

Either way, adopt a preventive approach to all the things you need to do and plan everything out. During the day, try to stay active and busy with tasks. This will keep your mind away from food and hunger. The first few times you carry out IF, you will feel hungry.

Remember that this isn't your body feeling hungry. It's simply a reaction to it expecting food at that point in time thanks to the way it has been conditioned. In other words, it's clock hunger and isn't real. You can try to drink some water at this time or have a cup of coffee to push it back. Over the course of a week, you'll find that your body will adjust to it and you'll be fine.

Use Coffee and Tea

When clock hunger strikes your best friends will be coffee and tea. Tea is an especially good choice, specifically green tea. Green tea is a great source of antioxidants and helps fight free radicals. Over and above this, drinking fluids helps reduce those hunger pangs that will occur during the first week when you're adopting IF.

Combine IF With Other Protocols

One of the best things you can do once you've adjusted to IF is to combine it with a low carb diet such as the ketogenic diet. This will help you lose fat a lot faster. Keep in mind that the keto diet is not an easy one to follow, especially for vegans. The best approach to take is to ease into it.

You can start off by following it on your rest days to see if you're able to make it work. If this is the case, you can expand it to your workout days. Your body will take some time to adjust to the keto diet and to be honest, the diet itself is the subject of an entire book and in the interest of space, I'll restrict myself to a few important points.

The first thing to remember with keto is that your body is going to take some time to adjust from burning carbs to fat. Remember that carbs are the primary source of fuel and your body isn't going to simply flip a switch and start burning fat. There is a transition period and this often referred to as the keto fog.

During this time, which lasts for a week or so, you will feel less energized and you'll feel as if you're not able to get out of second gear. The fog lasts for a week and once this time passes, your body will be able to burn fat as its primary source of fuel pretty easily. Practicing keto on your non-training days is a good way to get your body used to burning fat as its primary fuel source.

The best way to prepare for keto is to plan ahead of time and make sure your meal prep is on point. Always start with your protein intake and then move to the other macros. It is best to calculate your macros and calories upfront and then keep your meals as uniform as possible to help avoid calorie counting becoming overwhelming.

Ease yourself into keto much as you would with IF and you'll find that both protocols combined will make a massive difference to your overall health.

Do Not Binge

A common mistake beginners make is to look at the start of the feeding window as being a free for all as far as food is concerned. At first, this can be hard to resist since you'll look at the fasting period as being a wasteland without any food whatsoever. The reason this point of view develops is due to the fact that people think of IF as being restrictive.

When I say restrictive I mean to say that some people think of it as being a protocol where you deny yourself food for a period of time and need to use your willpower to stop yourself from eating. Here's the thing: Human beings are well designed to fast. Think of how our ancestors lived before we built cities and farms and gave birth to the Kardashians.

Food was scarce and wasn't guaranteed. After all, there isn't any deer in this world that will willingly offer itself up to be eaten. People had to go through periods where there wasn't any food available and they still managed to survive. As I've mentioned previously, we've come to associate the clock with our meal times and more often than not we feel clock hunger and not real hunger.

It's gotten to the point where some people don't even know what hunger feels like. IF is simply bringing you back into your natural eating pattern and is preventing you from going down the rabbit hole of allowing the clock to dictate what your stomach needs.

The other problem is with regards to breakfast. How often has someone wagged their finger at you and said, "Breakfast is the most important meal of the day!" Here's a fun fact for you: That saying was a marketing slogan invented by Kelloggs to sell more cereal. Here's another fun fact: John Harvey Kellogg the founder of the company figured breakfast was the solution to cure the sin of masturbation amongst young people (The Surprising Reason Why Dr. John Harvey Kellogg Invented Corn Flakes, 2020).

No, I'm not making that up! You can see his line of thought. You can't masturbate if you're shoving god awful cereal into your face, can you? Either way, that's the background story of the so called "most important meal of the day". There is no proof of any adverse effects of skipping breakfast or of not eating breakfast during the time designated for it (Leangains.com, 2020).

All in all, don't worry about skipping breakfast or even a meal. All that matters is your calories in versus out. Recognize what clock hunger is and get back in touch with your body's needs.

Exercise Tips

Here are some tips to make exercising and staying active easier for you. People think of exercise as being a chore and perhaps you're looking at it the same way.

Activity... Not Exercise

If you feel exercise is too darn painful for you to carry out regularly, make it a goal to be as active as possible. Walk as much as you can, climb a flight of stairs instead of taking the elevator and so on. Try lifting your grocery bags instead of using a cart to push them to your car and so on.

One of the best ways to start getting active is to find a community. Don't worry about joining gyms and so on in the beginning. As I mentioned earlier, just start moving and find someone to move with you. A great way to get fit is to join a salsa or a Zumba class where you'll meet other like-minded people and essentially con yourself into getting fit.

These classes only go so far though and once your body adjusts to it, you will need to join a gym to keep building your muscle mass. Again, you're not going to turn into the hulk. There are who knows how many millennia of evolution built into your body and genes and to think that a few weights will turn you into a man is absurd.

Joining a Crossfit Box (gym) is a great way of getting fit. The workout is planned for you and you're guaranteed a community that will support you in your fitness journey. It can be intimidating to join but once you do you'll find that the community aspect is Crossfit's best quality.

The workout will help you build muscle and lose fat and you'll also receive education from the trainers as to the best way to stay fit. In addition to this, one of the problems beginners face at the start is overtraining. Having an instructor around will prevent this from happening.

If you do join a regular gym by yourself, follow the starting strength program as mentioned earlier. This is a very well structured program that will guide you every step of the way. You'll always know where you stand so don't worry about getting lost.

Progressive Overload

Every exercise you do, remember the principle of progressive overload. This applies to activities that don't involve weights as well. Push yourself a little bit more every single time you perform the activity.

The biggest advantage, aside from better performance, is that you'll discover your boundaries easily. You'll learn how to listen to your body and be able to differentiate between laziness and genuine fatigue. Keep pushing yourself in this manner and your brain will get used to being uncomfortable and expand your limits.

Motivation

Everyone has bad days and there are sometimes when you just need a break from all of it. A break is a great idea but the problem is that most people don't know how to go about doing it at first. The best way to figure out if you need to take a step back is to adopt a 'do something' approach.

Let's say you return from work and don't feel like going to the gym. You feel exhausted and you feel mentally spent. Suit up and go to the gym anyway. Walk on the floor and try to go through your workout. For most beginners, these workouts will be amongst the best they'll ever have. Your brain will try to trick you using laziness and once you find that you can perform to your usual levels without any issues, you'll be energized and feel refreshed.

Then there are times when you'll find that you genuinely cannot perform the activity in question. In such cases, feel free to pack up and return home. Remember, discipline is great but being kind to yourself is the most important thing. I'm not talking about giving into laziness but to heed genuine concerns. If your body tells you it needs rest and if you confirm this need (via inadequate performance in the gym,) simply go home and call it a day.

Most beginners do the opposite. They give into laziness in the name of listening to their bodies and push through fatigue in the name of being motivated. You already know why you're getting into IF. The very fact that you're reading this book is an indication that you have all the motivation you need.

What you think of as a lack of motivation is temporary fatigue or laziness. As you become more experienced and learn to listen to your body, you'll differentiate between the two easily. At the start, do something and you'll understand the differences better.

Change it up!

Your body will get used to the activities you perform when you carry them out over time. Take a week's break from your regularly scheduled activities to perform something else. This will refresh your muscles and give them a different challenge to deal with. For example, if you're on Starting Strength and want to switch things up, suspend the program for a week.

Walk around the gym and hit the machines (which starting strength doesn't use). Instead of squatting as the program calls for you to do, perform some leg isolation exercises. Get creative! As long as you lift some weight and perform different exercises which target the same muscles, you'll be fine. You don't target each and every one but as long as you hit the majority of them, you'll be fine.

The benefit of doing this is that it will get your body used to moving in different ways and will make you stronger in more functional ways. This is over and above the mental benefit of feeling refreshed thanks to the novelty of doing something new. Lastly, it will prevent from falling into a fitness rut where you keep doing the same thing over and over again.

Remember, consistency and a rut are two very different things. The moment you find yourself becoming disillusioned, refresh yourself by doing something else for a week. When you get back to your usual routine, you'll appreciate it more.

Conclusion

Intermittent fasting is a great way to get fit and live a healthy life. As you've learned in this book, it's more of a lifestyle than it is a diet. While most diets are restrictive and require you to eliminate certain types of food, IF doesn't place any such restrictions on you. If anything, it helps you get back in touch with the way people used to eat.

The fact is that our bodies are well designed to incorporate fasts as you've learned. Therefore, you have nothing but the mental effects of clock base hunger to fear. As you observe yourself and become more aware of how this affects your perception of hunger, you'll realize that IF is a pretty easy protocol to follow.

The premise of it is simplicity itself. Fast for a certain amount of time and eat for another fixed amount of time. You can vary the size of these windows but the most common one is a 16/8 approach where you fast for 16 hours and eat during an eight-hour window.

A more complex approach is the Leangains method which requires you to count calories. As outlined in this book, you should seek to ease yourself into this approach if you've never done this before or if you find this intimidating. Start off with the Crescendo method and then move ahead as you get used to IF.

The key to succeeding with IF is to plan ahead of time and meal prepping and planning your recipes ahead of time is key. There is a one-week meal plan in this book and you can use it to create delicious meals for yourself. Make sure you've stocked up on the essentials as listed in here, this will make sure you always have something to create meals from.

Last but not least, remember that dieting and fat loss isn't rocket science. It is all about following a proven method. Don't worry about things like motivation etc. The changes you'll be making are small enough to cause close to no friction in your lifestyle and you'll find that IF is a great way to achieve your goals.

I wish you the best of luck on your journey! Let me know what you think of everything you've read and how this information has helped you!

References

A Brief History of USDA Food Guides. (2020). Retrieved 23 January 2020, from https://www.choosemyplate.gov/eathealthy/brief-history-usda-food-guides

Cotton, M. (2019). How Insulin Works with Glucose | Kaiser Permanente Washington. Retrieved 23 January 2020, from https://wa.kaiserpermanente.org/healthAndWellness/index .jhtml?item=%2Fcommon%2FhealthAndWellness%2Fcondit ions%2Fdiabetes%2FinsulinProcess.html

Coyle, D. (2018). Intermittent Fasting For Women: A Beginner's Guide. Retrieved 23 January 2020, from https://www.healthline.com/nutrition/intermittent-fasting-for-women

Hicks, C. (2016). Why fasting is now back in fashion. Retrieved 23 January 2020, from https://www.telegraph.co.uk/lifestyle/11524808/The-history-of-fasting.html

Hicks, D. (2018). Intermittent Fasting For Women: A Beginner's Guide. Retrieved 23 January 2020, from https://www.healthline.com/nutrition/intermittent-fasting-for-women#bottom-line

How Sugar Converts to Fat. (2020). Retrieved 23 January 2020, from https://healthcare.utah.edu/the-scope/shows.php?shows=0_7frg4jjd

Is The Sugar in Fruit Wrecking Your Diet?. (2020). Retrieved 23 January 2020, from https://nutritiouslife.com/eat-empowered/the-truth-about-fruit/

Kubala, J. (2018). The Warrior Diet: Review and Beginner's Guide. Retrieved 23 January 2020, from https://www.healthline.com/nutrition/warrior-diet-guide#bottom-line

Leangains.com. (2020). Retrieved 23 January 2020, from https://leangains.com/

Morin, A. (2019). The Effects of Childhood Trauma and What Can Help Alleviate Them. Retrieved 23 January 2020, from https://www.verywellmind.com/what-are-the-effects-of-childhood-trauma-4147640

Scott, J. (2019). What Is Calories In vs. Calories Out?. Retrieved 23 January 2020, from https://www.verywellfit.com/back-to-basics-the-reality-of-calories-3495603

The Surprising Reason Why Dr. John Harvey Kellogg Invented Corn Flakes. (2020). Retrieved 23 January 2020, from https://www.forbes.com/sites/priceonomics/2016/05/17/the-surprising-reason-why-dr-john-harvey-kellogg-invented-corn-flakes/#1fea4cbf6997